# 2. Scrambled Egg Whites with Spinach

## Ingredient:

• 4 egg whites
• 1 cup fresh spinach, chopped
• 1/4 teaspoon black pepper
• 1/4 teaspoon garlic powder
• 1/4 teaspoon onion powder
• 1 teaspoon olive oil

## Instructions:

1. In a bowl, whisk the egg whites until frothy.

2. Heat olive oil in a non•stick skillet over medium heat.

3. Add the chopped spinach to the skillet and sauté for a few minutes until wilted.

4. Pour the whisked egg whites over the spinach in the skillet.

5. Sprinkle black pepper, garlic powder, and onion powder over the eggs.

6. Cook, stirring occasionally, until the eggs are cooked through and scrambled.

7. Serve hot and enjoy!

This recipe is low in phosphorus and can be a good source of protein for a renal diet. As always, it's recommended to consult with a healthcare provider or a dietitian for personalized dietary advice tailored to individual health needs.

# 3. Low•Sodium English Muffin with Jam

**Ingredient:**

• 1 whole grain or low•sodium English muffin
• 1•2 tablespoons of low•sodium fruit jam or spread

**Instructions:**

1. Toast the English muffin until it reaches your desired level of crispiness.

2. Spread the low•sodium fruit jam or spread on top of the toasted English muffin.

3. Enjoy your low•sodium English muffin with jam as a quick and tasty breakfast or snack option.

This recipe is low in sodium, making it suitable for individuals following a low•sodium diet. It's always a good idea to check the nutrition labels on the English muffin and jam to ensure they are low in sodium or opt for low•sodium varieties.

Welcome to the ***"Renal Diet Cookbook for Seniors Over 60: Supporting Your Kidneys with Wholesome, Balanced Meals."*** This book is thoughtfully crafted to cater to the unique dietary needs of seniors managing kidney health. As we age, our bodies undergo various changes, and our nutritional requirements evolve. For those over 60, maintaining kidney health becomes increasingly crucial, and diet plays a significant role in this endeavor.

Kidney disease can be a daunting diagnosis, but with the right nutritional approach, it's possible to manage the condition effectively and maintain a high quality of life. This cookbook aims to empower you with the knowledge and recipes needed to support your kidney health through delicious, nutritious meals. Whether you are newly diagnosed or have been managing kidney disease for years, this book provides a wealth of information and culinary inspiration tailored specifically for seniors.

**In the following pages, you will find:**

- ***Understanding Kidney Health:*** An overview of kidney function, the impact of diet on kidney health, and key dietary considerations for those with renal concerns.

- ***Nutritional Guidance:*** Essential tips on managing sodium, potassium, phosphorus, and protein intake, along with other critical nutrients that affect kidney function.

- ***Meal Planning:*** Practical advice on creating balanced meal plans that support kidney health while catering to your taste preferences and lifestyle.

- ***Delicious Recipes:*** A diverse collection of recipes designed to be both kidney-friendly and flavorful. From hearty breakfasts to satisfying dinners, these recipes are easy to prepare and packed with nutrients.

- ***Lifestyle Tips:*** Additional advice on maintaining an active and healthy lifestyle, managing stress, and staying hydrated to support overall well-being.

Our recipes prioritize wholesome, natural ingredients to ensure you enjoy every bite while nourishing your body. Each recipe is carefully crafted to balance flavor and nutrition, making it easier to adhere to your renal diet without feeling deprived.

Living with kidney disease requires careful attention to your diet, but it doesn't mean you have to sacrifice enjoyment and variety in your meals. This cookbook is your companion in the kitchen, offering practical solutions and delicious recipes that help you thrive.

Thank you for choosing the ***"Renal Diet Cookbook for Seniors Over 60."*** Here's to your health, happiness, and culinary adventure!

# 1. Oatmeal with Blueberries and Cinnamon

**Ingredient:**

- 1/2 cup old·fashioned oats
- 1 cup water
- 1/4 cup fresh blueberries
- 1/2 teaspoon ground cinnamon
- 1 tablespoon chopped walnuts (optional)

**Instructions:**

1. In a small saucepan, bring water to a boil.

2. Stir in the oats and reduce heat to low. Cook for about 5 minutes, stirring occasionally, until the oats are cooked and the mixture thickens.

3. Remove the saucepan from heat and let it sit for a minute.

4. Stir in the blueberries and cinnamon.

5. Serve the oatmeal in a bowl and top with chopped walnuts if desired.

This recipe is low in sodium and phosphorus, making it suitable for a renal diet. It's important to consult with a healthcare provider or a dietitian for personalized dietary recommendations based on individual health needs.

# 4. Apple Cinnamon Pancakes

**Ingredient:**

- 1 cup all•purpose flour
- 1 tablespoon sugar
- 1 teaspoon baking powder
- 1/2 teaspoon baking soda
- 1/2 teaspoon ground cinnamon
- 1/4 teaspoon salt
- 1 cup buttermilk
- 1 large egg
- 2 tablespoons unsalted butter, melted
- 1 apple, peeled and diced
- Cooking spray or additional butter for cooking

**Instructions**:

1. In a mixing bowl, whisk together the flour, sugar, baking powder, baking soda, cinnamon, and salt.

2. In a separate bowl, whisk together the buttermilk, egg, and melted butter.

3. Pour the wet ingredients into the dry ingredients and stir until just combined. Do not overmix; it's okay if the batter is a bit lumpy.

4. Gently fold in the diced apple.

5. Heat a non•stick skillet or griddle over medium heat and lightly coat with cooking spray or butter.

6. Pour 1/4 cup of batter onto the skillet for each pancake.

7. Cook until bubbles form on the surface of the pancake, then flip and cook until golden brown on the other side.

8. Repeat with the remaining batter.Serve the apple cinnamon pancakes warm with a sprinkle of cinnamon on top.

These apple cinnamon pancakes are a flavorful and kidney•friendly breakfast option. It's always advisable to consult with a healthcare provider or a dietitian for personalized dietary recommendations based on individual health needs.

# 5. Greek Yogurt with Strawberries and Honey

**Ingredient:**

• 1/2 cup plain Greek yogurt (low•fat or non•fat)
• 1/2 cup fresh strawberries, sliced
• 1 tablespoon honey
• 1 tablespoon chopped nuts (optional)

**Instructions**:

1. In a bowl, place the Greek yogurt.

2. Top the yogurt with the sliced strawberries.

3. Drizzle the honey over the strawberries.

4. Sprinkle chopped nuts on top if desired for added texture and flavor.

5. Enjoy this nutritious and delicious Greek yogurt with strawberries and honey as a healthy breakfast or snack option.

This recipe is low in sodium and phosphorus, making it suitable for a renal diet. It's important to consult with a healthcare provider or a dietitian for personalized dietary recommendations tailored to individual health needs.

# 6. Quinoa Porridge with Almond Milk and Maple Syrup

**Ingredient:**

• 1/2 cup quinoa, rinsed
• 1 cup unsweetened almond milk
• 1/2 teaspoon ground cinnamon
• 1/4 teaspoon vanilla extract
• 1 tablespoon pure maple syrup
• 1 tablespoon chopped almonds (optional)

**Instructions:**

1. In a saucepan, combine the quinoa and almond milk.

2. Bring the mixture to a boil, then reduce heat to low and simmer for about 15•20 minutes, stirring occasionally, until the quinoa is cooked and the mixture thickens.

3. Stir in the ground cinnamon and vanilla extract.

4. Remove the saucepan from heat and let it sit for a minute.

5. Drizzle the maple syrup over the quinoa porridge.

6. Serve the quinoa porridge in a bowl and top with chopped almonds if desired.

This recipe is low in sodium and phosphorus, making it suitable for a renal diet. It's important to consult with a healthcare provider or a dietitian for personalized dietary recommendations based on individual health needs.

# 7. Banana Nut Muffins (Low Potassium)

**Ingredient:**

- 1 cup all•purpose flour
- 1/2 cup granulated sugar
- 1 teaspoon baking powder
- 1/2 teaspoon baking soda
- 1/4 teaspoon salt
- 2 ripe bananas, mashed
- 1/4 cup unsalted butter, melted
- 1/4 cup chopped walnuts
- 1/2 teaspoon vanilla extract
- 1 large egg

**Instructions:**

1. Preheat the oven to 350°F (175°C) and line a muffin tin with paper liners.

2. In a mixing bowl, whisk together the flour, sugar, baking powder, baking soda, and salt.

3. In a separate bowl, mix the mashed bananas, melted butter, vanilla extract, and egg.

4. Combine the wet ingredients with the dry ingredients and stir until just combined.

5. Gently fold in the chopped walnuts.

6. Spoon the batter into the muffin cups, filling each about 2/3 full.

7. Bake for 18•20 minutes or until a toothpick inserted into the center of a muffin comes out clean.

8. Allow the muffins to cool in the pan for a few minutes before transferring them to a wire rack to cool completely.

These Banana Nut Muffins are low in potassium and can be a delicious treat for those following a renal diet. It's always best to consult with a healthcare provider or a dietitian for personalized dietary recommendations based on individual health needs.

# 8. Rice Cakes with Peanut Butter

**Ingredient:**

• 2 rice cakes (low•sodium if available)
• 2 tablespoons natural peanut butter (unsalted)
• 1 small banana, sliced
• Cinnamon (optional)

**Instructions**:
1. Spread 1 tablespoon of peanut butter on each rice cake.

2. Top the peanut butter with sliced banana.

3. Sprinkle a little cinnamon on top if desired for extra flavor.

4. Enjoy your rice cakes with peanut butter and banana as a kidney•friendly snack or light meal option.

This recipe is low in sodium and phosphorus, making it suitable for a renal diet. It's important to consult with a healthcare provider or a dietitian for personalized dietary recommendations based on individual health needs.

# 9. Cottage Cheese with Pineapple

**Ingredient:**

• 1/2 cup low•fat cottage cheese
• 1/2 cup fresh pineapple chunks
• 1 tablespoon chopped walnuts (optional)

**Instructions:**

1. In a bowl, place the low•fat cottage cheese.

2. Top the cottage cheese with fresh pineapple chunks.

3. Sprinkle chopped walnuts on top if desired for added texture and flavor.

4. Enjoy this nutritious and delicious cottage cheese with pineapple as a healthy snack or light meal option.

This recipe is low in sodium and phosphorus, making it suitable for a renal diet. It's important to consult with a healthcare provider or a dietitian for personalized dietary recommendations tailored to individual health needs.

# 10. Breakfast Smoothie (Berries, Almond Milk, Spinach)

**Ingredient:**

• 1/2 cup mixed berries (such as strawberries, blueberries, raspberries)
• 1 cup unsweetened almond milk
• 1 cup fresh spinach leaves
• 1 tablespoon chia seeds (optional)
• 1 tablespoon honey (optional)

**Instructions:**

1. In a blender, combine the mixed berries, almond milk, fresh spinach leaves, and chia seeds.

2. Blend until smooth and well combined.

3. Taste the smoothie and add honey if desired for sweetness.

4. Pour the smoothie into a glass and enjoy this nutritious and kidney•friendly breakfast option.

This smoothie is low in sodium and phosphorus, making it suitable for a renal diet. It's important to consult with a healthcare provider or a dietitian for personalized dietary recommendations based on individual health needs.

# 11. Egg White Omelet with Bell Peppers and Onions

**Ingredient:**

- 4 egg whites
- 1/4 cup diced bell peppers (any color)
- 1/4 cup diced onions
- 1/4 teaspoon black pepper
- 1/4 teaspoon garlic powder
- 1/4 teaspoon onion powder
- 1 teaspoon olive oil

**Instructions:**

1. In a bowl, whisk the egg whites until frothy.

2. Heat olive oil in a non•stick skillet over medium heat.

3. Add the diced bell peppers and onions to the skillet and sauté until they are softened.

4. Pour the whisked egg whites over the sautéed vegetables in the skillet.

5. Sprinkle black pepper, garlic powder, and onion powder over the eggs.

6. Cook, stirring occasionally, until the eggs are cooked through and the omelet is set.
7. Fold the omelet in half and slide it onto a plate.

8. Serve hot and enjoy this kidney•friendly Egg White Omelet with Bell Peppers and Onions.

This recipe is low in sodium and phosphorus, making it suitable for a renal diet. It's important to consult with a healthcare provider or a dietitian for personalized dietary recommendations based on individual health needs.

# 12. Whole Wheat Toast with Avocado Spread

## Ingredient:

• 1 ripe avocado
• 2 slices of whole wheat bread, toasted
• 1/4 teaspoon black pepper
• 1/4 teaspoon garlic powder
• 1/4 teaspoon onion powder
• 1 teaspoon lemon juice
• Pinch of salt (optional)

## Instructions:

1. In a bowl, mash the ripe avocado with a fork until smooth.

2. Add black pepper, garlic powder, onion powder, lemon juice, and salt (if using) to the mashed avocado and mix well.

3. Spread the avocado mixture on top of the toasted whole wheat bread slices.

4. Serve the Whole Wheat Toast with Avocado Spread as a kidney•friendly and nutritious breakfast or snack option.

This recipe is low in sodium and phosphorus, making it suitable for a renal diet. It's important to consult with a healthcare provider or a dietitian for personalized dietary recommendations based on individual health needs.

# 13. Lemon Poppy Seed Muffins

**Ingredient:**

- 1 1/2 cups all•purpose flour
- 1/2 cup granulated sugar
- 2 tablespoons poppy seeds
- 1 tablespoon lemon zest
- 1 teaspoon baking powder
- 1/2 teaspoon baking soda
- 1/4 teaspoon salt
- 1/2 cup unsweetened applesauce
- 1/4 cup fresh lemon juice
- 1/4 cup low•fat milk
- 1/4 cup vegetable oil
- 1 large egg

**Instructions:**

1. Preheat the oven to 375°F (190°C) and line a muffin tin with paper liners.

2. In a mixing bowl, whisk together the flour, sugar, poppy seeds, lemon zest, baking powder, baking soda, and salt.

3. In a separate bowl, mix the applesauce, lemon juice, milk, vegetable oil, and egg.

4. Combine the wet ingredients with the dry ingredients and stir until just combined.

5. Spoon the batter into the muffin cups, filling each about 2/3 full.

6. Bake for 18•20 minutes or until a toothpick inserted into the center of a muffin comes out clean.

7. Allow the muffins to cool in the pan for a few minutes before transferring them to a wire rack to cool completely.

These Lemon Poppy Seed Muffins are low in sodium and phosphorus, making them suitable for a renal diet. It's always best to consult with a healthcare provider or a dietitian for personalized dietary recommendations based on individual health needs.

# 14. French Toast with Fresh Berries

**Ingredient:**

• 2 slices of whole wheat bread
• 2 large eggs
• 1/4 cup low•fat milk
• 1/2 teaspoon ground cinnamon
• 1/2 teaspoon vanilla extract
• Cooking spray
• Fresh berries (such as strawberries, blueberries, raspberries) for topping
• Sugar•free syrup (optional)

**Instructions:**

1. In a shallow dish, whisk together the eggs, low•fat milk, ground cinnamon, and vanilla extract.

2. Dip each slice of whole wheat bread into the egg mixture, making sure to coat both sides.

3. Heat a non•stick skillet over medium heat and lightly coat with cooking spray.

4. Cook the dipped bread slices in the skillet until golden brown on both sides.

5. Serve the French toast topped with fresh berries and a drizzle of sugar•free syrup if desired.

This French Toast with Fresh Berries recipe is low in sodium and phosphorus, making it suitable for a renal diet. It's important to consult with a healthcare provider or a dietitian for personalized dietary recommendations based on individual health needs.

# 15. Cream of Wheat with Brown Sugar and Butter

**Ingredient:**

• 1/4 cup Cream of Wheat
• 1 cup water
• 1 tablespoon brown sugar
• 1 teaspoon unsalted butter

**Instructions:**

1. In a small saucepan, bring water to a boil.

2. Slowly whisk in the Cream of Wheat and reduce heat to low.

3. Cook for about 2•3 minutes, stirring occasionally, until the mixture thickens.

4. Remove from heat and let it sit for a minute to cool slightly.

5. Stir in the brown sugar and unsalted butter until well combined.

6. Serve the Cream of Wheat in a bowl and enjoy this kidney•friendly breakfast option.

It's important to consult with a healthcare provider or a dietitian for personalized dietary recommendations tailored to individual health needs, including for those following a renal diet.

# 16. Low•Sodium Turkey Sausage and Egg White Breakfast Burrito

## Ingredient:

• 2 low•sodium turkey sausage links, chopped
• 2 egg whites
• 1 whole wheat tortilla
• 1/4 cup diced bell peppers
• 1/4 cup diced onions
• 1/4 teaspoon black pepper
• 1/4 teaspoon garlic powder
• 1/4 teaspoon onion powder
• 1 teaspoon olive oil

## Instructions:

1. In a skillet, heat olive oil over medium heat.

2. Add the chopped turkey sausage links, diced bell peppers, and onions to the skillet and sauté until the vegetables are tender and the sausage is cooked.

3. In a separate bowl, whisk the egg whites with black pepper, garlic powder, and onion powder.

4. Push the sausage and vegetable mixture to one side of the skillet and pour the egg whites into the other side.

5. Cook the egg whites, stirring occasionally, until they are scrambled and cooked through.

6. Warm the whole wheat tortilla in the skillet or microwave.

7. Place the cooked egg whites, turkey sausage, and vegetable mixture in the center of the tortilla.

8. Roll up the tortilla to form a burrito. Serve the Low•Sodium Turkey Sausage and Egg White Breakfast Burrito as a kidney•friendly and nutritious breakfast option.

This recipe is low in sodium and can be a good source of protein for a renal diet. It's important to consult with a healthcare provider or a dietitian for personalized dietary recommendations based on individual health needs.

# 17. Almond Milk Chia Seed Pudding

**Ingredient:**

- 1/4 cup chia seeds
- 1 cup unsweetened almond milk
- 1/2 teaspoon vanilla extract
- 1 tablespoon honey or maple syrup (optional)
- Fresh berries for topping

**Instructions:**

1. In a bowl, mix together chia seeds, almond milk, vanilla extract, and honey or maple syrup (if using).

2. Stir well to combine all ingredients.

3. Cover the bowl and refrigerate for at least 2 hours or overnight to allow the chia seeds to absorb the liquid and thicken.

4. Stir the mixture again before serving to ensure a pudding•like consistency.

5. Serve the Almond Milk Chia Seed Pudding topped with fresh berries.

This recipe is low in sodium and phosphorus, making it suitable for a renal diet. It's important to consult with a healthcare provider or a dietitian for personalized dietary recommendations based on individual health needs.

# 18. Berry Parfait with Greek Yogurt

## Ingredient:

• 1/2 cup mixed berries (such as strawberries, blueberries, raspberries)
• 1/2 cup low•fat Greek yogurt
• 1 tablespoon chopped nuts (such as almonds or walnuts)
• 1 tablespoon honey (optional)

## Instructions:

1. In a glass or bowl, layer half of the Greek yogurt at the bottom.

2. Add a layer of mixed berries on top of the yogurt.

3. Repeat with another layer of Greek yogurt and mixed berries.

4. Top the parfait with chopped nuts and drizzle honey on top if desired.

5. Serve the Berry Parfait with Greek Yogurt as a kidney•friendly and nutritious breakfast or snack option.

This recipe is low in sodium and phosphorus, making it suitable for a renal diet. It's important to consult with a healthcare provider or a dietitian for personalized dietary recommendations based on individual health needs.

# 19. Low•Sodium Waffles with Fresh Fruit

## Ingredient:

• 1 cup all•purpose flour
• 1 tablespoon sugar
• 1 teaspoon baking powder
• 1/2 teaspoon baking soda
• 1/4 teaspoon salt
• 1 cup low•fat buttermilk
• 1 large egg
• 1 tablespoon unsalted butter, melted
• Cooking spray
• Fresh fruit for topping (such as berries, sliced bananas)

## Instructions:

1. In a mixing bowl, whisk together the flour, sugar, baking powder, baking soda, and salt.

2. In a separate bowl, mix the low•fat buttermilk, egg, and melted butter.

3. Combine the wet ingredients with the dry ingredients and stir until just combined.

4. Preheat a waffle iron and lightly coat with cooking spray.

5. Pour the batter onto the waffle iron and cook according to the manufacturer's instructions until golden brown.

6. Serve the Low•Sodium Waffles with Fresh Fruit as a kidney•friendly and delicious breakfast option, topped with fresh fruit.

This recipe is low in sodium and phosphorus, making it suitable for a renal diet. It's important to consult with a healthcare provider or a dietitian for personalized dietary recommendations based on individual health needs.

# 20. Pumpkin Spice Oatmeal

## Ingredient:

• 1/2 cup old•fashioned oats
• 1 cup water
• 1/4 cup canned pumpkin puree
• 1/2 teaspoon pumpkin pie spice
• 1 tablespoon chopped pecans or walnuts
• 1 tablespoon maple syrup (optional)

## Instructions:

1. In a small saucepan, bring water to a boil.

2. Stir in the oats and reduce heat to low. Cook for about 5 minutes, stirring occasionally, until the oats are cooked and the mixture thickens.

3. Stir in the canned pumpkin puree and pumpkin pie spice.

4. Cook for an additional 2•3 minutes, stirring occasionally.

5. Remove the saucepan from heat and let it sit for a minute.

6. Serve the Pumpkin Spice Oatmeal in a bowl and top with chopped pecans or walnuts.

7. Drizzle with maple syrup if desired for added sweetness.

This recipe is low in sodium and phosphorus, making it suitable for a renal diet. It's important to consult with a healthcare provider or a dietitian for personalized dietary recommendations based on individual health needs.

# 21. Grilled Chicken Salad with Low•Sodium Dressing

**Ingredient:**

• 4 oz grilled chicken breast, sliced
• Mixed salad greens (such as spinach, arugula, romaine)
• 1/4 cup cherry tomatoes, halved
• 1/4 cup cucumber, sliced
• 1/4 cup bell peppers, sliced
• 1/4 cup red onion, thinly sliced
• Low•sodium salad dressing of choice

**Instructions**:

1. In a large bowl, combine the mixed salad greens, cherry tomatoes, cucumber, bell peppers, and red onion.

2. Top the salad with the sliced grilled chicken breast.

3. Drizzle the low•sodium salad dressing over the salad.

4. Toss the salad gently to coat all ingredients with the dressing.

5. Serve the Grilled Chicken Salad with Low•Sodium Dressing as a kidney•friendly and nutritious meal option.

This recipe is low in sodium and phosphorus, making it suitable for a renal diet. It's important to consult with a healthcare provider or a dietitian for personalized dietary recommendations based on individual health needs.

# 22. Tuna Salad with Greek Yogurt

**Ingredient:**

• 1 can (5 oz) tuna in water, drained
• 1/4 cup low•fat Greek yogurt
• 1 tablespoon lemon juice
• 1/4 cup diced celery
• 1/4 cup diced red onion
• 1/4 teaspoon black pepper
• Lettuce leaves for serving

**Instructions**:

1. In a mixing bowl, combine the drained tuna, low•fat Greek yogurt, lemon juice, diced celery, diced red onion, and black pepper.

2. Mix well until all ingredients are evenly combined.

3. Serve the tuna salad on a bed of lettuce leaves or as a sandwich filling.

4. Enjoy this kidney•friendly Tuna Salad with Greek Yogurt as a nutritious meal option.

This recipe is low in sodium and phosphorus, making it suitable for a renal diet. It's important to consult with a healthcare provider or a dietitian for personalized dietary recommendations based on individual health needs.

# 23. Turkey and Avocado Wrap

## Ingredient:

- 4 oz sliced turkey breast
- 1/4 avocado, sliced
- 1 whole wheat or low•sodium wrap
- 1/4 cup shredded lettuce
- 1/4 cup diced tomatoes
- Mustard or low•sodium mayonnaise (optional)

## Instructions:

1. Lay the whole wheat or low•sodium wrap flat on a clean surface.

2. Layer the sliced turkey breast, avocado slices, shredded lettuce, and diced tomatoes on the wrap.

3. Add a spread of mustard or low•sodium mayonnaise if desired.

4. Roll up the wrap tightly, tucking in the sides as you go.

5. Slice the wrap in half diagonally for easier eating.

6. Serve the Turkey and Avocado Wrap as a kidney•friendly and nutritious meal option.

This recipe is low in sodium and phosphorus, making it suitable for a renal diet. It's important to consult with a healthcare provider or a dietitian for personalized dietary recommendations based on individual health needs.

# 24. Quinoa Salad with Cucumber and Tomato

**Ingredient:**

• 1 cup quinoa, rinsed
• 2 cups water
• 1 cucumber, diced
• 1 cup cherry tomatoes, halved
• 1/4 cup chopped fresh parsley
• 1/4 cup diced red onion
• 2 tablespoons olive oil
• 2 tablespoons lemon juice
• Salt and pepper to taste

**Instructions:**

1. In a saucepan, bring the water to a boil. Add the quinoa, reduce heat to low, cover, and simmer for about 15 minutes or until the quinoa is cooked and the water is absorbed. Remove from heat and let it cool.

2. In a large bowl, combine the cooked quinoa, diced cucumber, cherry tomatoes, chopped parsley, and diced red onion.

3. In a small bowl, whisk together the olive oil, lemon juice, salt, and pepper to make the dressing.

4. Pour the dressing over the quinoa salad and toss to combine.

5. Adjust seasoning if needed and chill in the refrigerator before serving.

6. Serve the Quinoa Salad with Cucumber and Tomato as a kidney•friendly and nutritious side dish or light meal option.

This recipe is low in sodium and phosphorus, making it suitable for a renal diet. It's important to consult with a healthcare provider or a dietitian for personalized dietary recommendations based on individual health needs.

# 25. Low•Sodium Chicken Noodle Soup

**Ingredient:**

• 4 cups low•sodium chicken broth
• 1 cup cooked chicken breast, shredded
• 1 carrot, sliced
• 1 celery stalk, sliced
• 1/2 cup diced onion
• 1 garlic clove, minced
• 1/2 cup uncooked egg noodles
• 1/2 teaspoon dried thyme
• Salt•free seasoning blend to taste
• Chopped fresh parsley for garnish

**Instructions:**

1. In a large pot, bring the low•sodium chicken broth to a simmer over medium heat.

2. Add the cooked chicken breast, carrot, celery, onion, and garlic to the pot.

3. Simmer for about 10•15 minutes until the vegetables are tender.

4. Add the uncooked egg noodles and dried thyme to the pot and cook according to the package instructions for the noodles.

5. Season the soup with salt•free seasoning blend to taste.

6. Serve the Low•Sodium Chicken Noodle Soup hot, garnished with chopped fresh parsley.

This recipe is low in sodium and phosphorus, making it suitable for a renal diet. It's important to consult with a healthcare provider or a dietitian for personalized dietary recommendations based on individual health needs.

# 26. Spinach and Strawberry Salad with Walnuts

**Ingredient:**

• 2 cups fresh spinach leaves
• 1/2 cup sliced strawberries
• 2 tablespoons chopped walnuts
• 1 tablespoon balsamic vinegar
• 1 tablespoon olive oil
• 1 teaspoon honey
• Salt and pepper to taste

**Instructions:**

1. In a large bowl, combine the fresh spinach leaves, sliced strawberries, and chopped walnuts.

2. In a small bowl, whisk together the balsamic vinegar, olive oil, honey, salt, and pepper to make the dressing.

3. Drizzle the dressing over the spinach, strawberry, and walnut mixture.

4. Toss the salad gently to coat all ingredients with the dressing.

5. Serve the Spinach and Strawberry Salad with Walnuts as a kidney•friendly and nutritious meal option.

This recipe is low in sodium and phosphorus, making it suitable for a renal diet. It's important to consult with a healthcare provider or a dietitian for personalized dietary recommendations based on individual health needs.

# 27. Veggie Wrap with Hummus

**Ingredient:**

- 1 whole wheat or low•sodium wrap
- 2 tablespoons hummus
- 1/4 cup shredded lettuce
- 1/4 cup sliced cucumber
- 1/4 cup sliced bell peppers
- 1/4 cup shredded carrots
- 1/4 cup diced tomatoes
- 1/4 cup diced red onion

**Instructions:**

1. Lay the whole wheat or low•sodium wrap flat on a clean surface.

2. Spread the hummus evenly over the wrap.

3. Layer the shredded lettuce, sliced cucumber, sliced bell peppers, shredded carrots, diced tomatoes, and diced red onion on top of the hummus.

4. Roll up the wrap tightly, tucking in the sides as you go.

5. Slice the wrap in half diagonally for easier eating.

6. Serve the Veggie Wrap with Hummus as a kidney•friendly and nutritious meal option.

This recipe is low in sodium and phosphorus, making it suitable for a renal diet. It's important to consult with a healthcare provider or a dietitian for personalized dietary recommendations based on individual health needs.

# 28. Grilled Shrimp Salad with Lemon Vinaigrette

**Ingredient:**

• 8 oz grilled shrimp
• Mixed salad greens (such as arugula, spinach, romaine)
• 1/4 cup cherry tomatoes, halved
• 1/4 cup cucumber, sliced
• 1/4 cup red onion, thinly sliced
• Lemon Vinaigrette:
  • 2 tablespoons olive oil
  • 1 tablespoon fresh lemon juice
  • 1 teaspoon Dijon mustard
  • Salt and pepper to taste

**Instructions:**

1. In a large bowl, combine the mixed salad greens, cherry tomatoes, cucumber, and red onion.

2. Top the salad with the grilled shrimp.

3. In a small bowl, whisk together the olive oil, lemon juice, Dijon mustard, salt, and pepper to make the vinaigrette.

4. Drizzle the lemon vinaigrette over the salad and shrimp.

5. Toss the salad gently to coat all ingredients with the vinaigrette.

6. Serve the Grilled Shrimp Salad with Lemon Vinaigrette as a kidney•friendly and nutritious meal option.

This recipe is low in sodium and phosphorus, making it suitable for a renal diet. It's important to consult with a healthcare provider or a dietitian for personalized dietary recommendations based on individual health needs.

# 29. Chickpea Salad with Cucumber and Mint

## Ingredient:

- 1 can (15 oz) chickpeas, drained and rinsed
- 1 cucumber, diced
- 1/4 cup red onion, finely chopped
- 2 tablespoons fresh mint leaves, chopped
- 2 tablespoons olive oil
- 2 tablespoons lemon juice
- Salt and pepper to taste

## Instructions:

1. In a large bowl, combine the chickpeas, diced cucumber, chopped red onion, and chopped mint leaves.

2. In a small bowl, whisk together the olive oil, lemon juice, salt, and pepper to make the dressing.

3. Pour the dressing over the chickpea salad and toss to combine.

4. Adjust seasoning if needed and chill in the refrigerator before serving.

5. Serve the Chickpea Salad with Cucumber and Mint as a kidney•friendly and nutritious side dish or light meal option.

This recipe is low in sodium and phosphorus, making it suitable for a renal diet. It's important to consult with a healthcare provider or a dietitian for personalized dietary recommendations based on individual health needs.

# 30. Roasted Vegetable Sandwich

**Ingredient:**

• 1 zucchini, sliced
• 1 yellow squash, sliced
• 1 red bell pepper, sliced
• 1 red onion, sliced
• 2 tablespoons olive oil
• Salt and pepper to taste
• Whole grain bread or low•sodium bread
• Hummus for spreading
• Fresh basil leaves

**Instructions**:

1. Preheat the oven to 400°F (200°C).

2. In a large bowl, toss the sliced zucchini, yellow squash, red bell pepper, and red onion with olive oil, salt, and pepper.

3. Spread the vegetables in a single layer on a baking sheet.

4. Roast the vegetables in the preheated oven for about 20•25 minutes or until they are tender and slightly caramelized.

5. Toast the whole grain bread or low•sodium bread slices.

6. Spread hummus on one side of the bread slices.

7. Layer the roasted vegetables on top of the hummus.

8. Top with fresh basil leaves and cover with another slice of bread to make a sandwich.

9. Serve the Roasted Vegetable Sandwich as a kidney•friendly and nutritious meal option.

This recipe is low in sodium and phosphorus, making it suitable for a renal diet. It's important to consult with a healthcare provider or a dietitian for personalized dietary recommendations based on individual health needs.

# 31. Turkey Burger with Whole Wheat Bun

**Ingredient:**

• 4 oz ground turkey
• 1/4 teaspoon garlic powder
• 1/4 teaspoon onion powder
• 1/4 teaspoon black pepper
• 1 whole wheat bun
• Lettuce, tomato slices, and onion slices for topping
• Mustard or low•sodium ketchup (optional)

**Instructions:**

1. In a bowl, mix the ground turkey with garlic powder, onion powder, and black pepper.
2. Form the seasoned turkey into a patty shape.

3. Grill or cook the turkey burger patty until fully cooked.

4. Toast the whole wheat bun.

5. Place the cooked turkey burger patty on the bottom half of the bun.

6. Top with lettuce, tomato slices, and onion slices.

7. Add mustard or low•sodium ketchup if desired.

8. Cover with the top half of the bun to complete the burger.

9. Serve the Turkey Burger with Whole Wheat Bun as a kidney•friendly and nutritious meal option.

This recipe is low in sodium and phosphorus, making it suitable for a renal diet. It's important to consult with a healthcare provider or a dietitian for personalized dietary recommendations based on individual health needs.

# 32. Lentil Soup with Carrots and Celery

## Ingredient:

• 1 cup dried lentils, rinsed
• 4 cups low•sodium vegetable or chicken broth
• 1 carrot, diced
• 1 celery stalk, diced
• 1/2 onion, diced
• 1 garlic clove, minced
• 1/2 teaspoon dried thyme
• Salt and pepper to taste
• Fresh parsley for garnish

## Instructions:

1. In a large pot, combine the dried lentils, low•sodium broth, carrot, celery, onion, garlic, and dried thyme.

2. Bring the mixture to a boil, then reduce heat to low and simmer for about 30•40 minutes or until the lentils are tender.

3. Season the soup with salt and pepper to taste.

4. Serve the Lentil Soup with Carrots and Celery hot, garnished with fresh parsley.

This recipe is low in sodium and phosphorus, making it suitable for a renal diet. It's important to consult with a healthcare provider or a dietitian for personalized dietary recommendations based on individual health needs.

# 33. Chicken and Apple Salad

**Ingredient:**

• 4 oz cooked chicken breast, diced
• 1 medium apple, diced
• 1/4 cup celery, diced
• 1/4 cup red onion, diced
• 2 tablespoons chopped walnuts
• 1/4 cup low•fat Greek yogurt
• 1 tablespoon lemon juice
• 1/4 teaspoon black pepper
• Lettuce leaves for serving

**Instructions:**

1. In a mixing bowl, combine the diced chicken breast, diced apple, diced celery, diced red onion, and chopped walnuts.

2. In a separate small bowl, mix the low•fat Greek yogurt, lemon juice, and black pepper to make the dressing.

3. Pour the dressing over the chicken and apple mixture and toss until well coated.

4. Serve the Chicken and Apple Salad on a bed of lettuce leaves or as a sandwich filling.

5. Enjoy this kidney•friendly Chicken and Apple Salad as a nutritious meal option.

This recipe is low in sodium and phosphorus, making it suitable for a renal diet. It's important to consult with a healthcare provider or a dietitian for personalized dietary recommendations based on individual health needs.

# 34. Low•Sodium Minestrone Soup

**Ingredient:**

• 1 tablespoon olive oil
• 1/2 cup diced onion
• 1/2 cup diced carrots
• 1/2 cup diced celery
• 2 cloves garlic, minced
• 4 cups low•sodium vegetable broth
• 1 can (15 oz) low•sodium diced tomatoes
• 1 can (15 oz) low•sodium kidney beans, drained and rinsed
• 1/2 cup small pasta (such as ditalini or small shells)
• 1 teaspoon dried basil
• 1 teaspoon dried oregano
• Salt and pepper to taste
• Fresh parsley for garnish

**Instructions**:

1. In a large pot, heat olive oil over medium heat.

2. Add diced onion, carrots, celery, and garlic. Cook until vegetables are tender, about 5•7 minutes.

3. Pour in the low•sodium vegetable broth and diced tomatoes. Bring to a simmer.

4. Add the drained and rinsed kidney beans, small pasta, dried basil, and dried oregano. Simmer for about 10•15 minutes or until the pasta is cooked.

5. Season with salt and pepper to taste.

6. Serve the Low•Sodium Minestrone Soup hot, garnished with fresh parsley.

This recipe is low in sodium and phosphorus, making it suitable for a renal diet. It's important to consult with a healthcare provider or a dietitian for personalized dietary recommendations based on individual health needs.

# 35. Roast Beef and Arugula Sandwich

**Ingredient:**

- 4 oz lean roast beef, thinly sliced
- Whole grain bread or low•sodium bread
- 1/2 cup arugula
- 1/4 cup sliced red onion
- 1/4 cup sliced tomato
- Mustard or low•sodium mayonnaise (optional)

**Instructions:**

1. Toast the whole grain bread or low•sodium bread slices.

2. Layer the thinly sliced roast beef on one slice of bread.

3. Top with arugula, sliced red onion, and sliced tomato.

4. Add mustard or low•sodium mayonnaise if desired.

5. Cover with the other slice of bread to complete the sandwich.

6. Serve the Roast Beef and Arugula Sandwich as a kidney•friendly and nutritious meal option.

This recipe is low in sodium and phosphorus, making it suitable for a renal diet. It's important to consult with a healthcare provider or a dietitian for personalized dietary recommendations based on individual health needs.

# 36. Egg Salad with Greek Yogurt on Whole Wheat Bread

**Ingredient:**

• 4 hard•boiled eggs, chopped
• 1/4 cup plain Greek yogurt
• 1 tablespoon Dijon mustard
• 1/4 cup diced celery
• 1/4 cup diced red onion
• Salt and pepper to taste
• Whole wheat bread or low•sodium bread
• Lettuce leaves for serving

**Instructions**:

1. In a bowl, combine the chopped hard•boiled eggs, plain Greek yogurt, Dijon mustard, diced celery, and diced red onion.

2. Mix well until all ingredients are evenly combined.

3. Season the egg salad with salt and pepper to taste.

4. Toast the whole wheat bread or low•sodium bread slices.

5. Place lettuce leaves on one slice of bread.

6. Top with the egg salad mixture.

7. Cover with another slice of bread to make a sandwich.

8. Serve the Egg Salad with Greek Yogurt on Whole Wheat Bread as a kidney•friendly and nutritious meal option.

This recipe is low in sodium and phosphorus, making it suitable for a renal diet. It's important to consult with a healthcare provider or a dietitian for personalized dietary recommendations based on individual health needs.

# 37. Mediterranean Quinoa Bowl

## Ingredient:

• 1 cup quinoa, rinsed
• 2 cups low•sodium vegetable broth
• 1 can (15 oz) chickpeas, drained and rinsed
• 1 cucumber, diced
• 1 cup cherry tomatoes, halved
• 1/4 cup red onion, finely chopped
• 1/4 cup Kalamata olives, sliced
• 1/4 cup crumbled feta cheese
• 2 tablespoons olive oil
• 2 tablespoons lemon juice
• 1 teaspoon dried oregano
• Salt and pepper to taste

## Instructions:

1. In a saucepan, bring the low•sodium vegetable broth to a boil. Add the quinoa, reduce heat to low, cover, and simmer for about 15 minutes or until the quinoa is cooked and the liquid is absorbed. Remove from heat and let it cool.

2. In a large bowl, combine the cooked quinoa, chickpeas, diced cucumber, cherry tomatoes, red onion, Kalamata olives, and crumbled feta cheese.

3. In a small bowl, whisk together the olive oil, lemon juice, dried oregano, salt, and pepper to make the dressing.

4. Pour the dressing over the quinoa salad and toss to combine.

5. Adjust seasoning if needed and chill in the refrigerator before serving.

6. Serve the Mediterranean Quinoa Bowl as a kidney•friendly and nutritious meal option.

This recipe is low in sodium and phosphorus, making it suitable for a renal diet. It's important to consult with a healthcare provider or a dietitian for personalized dietary recommendations based on individual health needs.

# 38. Avocado and Turkey Club

**Ingredient:**

• 2 slices whole wheat bread (low•sodium if possible)
• 1/4 ripe avocado, mashed
• 2 oz. low•sodium turkey breast slices
• 1/2 small tomato, sliced
• 1/4 cup baby spinach leaves
• 1 teaspoon low•sodium mayonnaise
• 1 teaspoon Dijon mustard
• Salt and pepper to taste

**Instructions:**
1. Toast the whole wheat bread slices until golden brown.

2. Spread the mashed avocado on one side of each bread slice.

3. Layer the turkey breast slices, tomato slices, and baby spinach leaves on one bread slice.

4. Spread the low•sodium mayonnaise and Dijon mustard on the other bread slice.

5. Season with salt and pepper to taste.

6. Close the sandwich by placing the mayo•mustard side on top of the turkey•veggie side.

7. Cut the sandwich in half diagonally and serve.

This recipe is kidney•friendly and suitable for seniors over 60 following a renal diet. Enjoy your Avocado and Turkey Club sandwich!

# 39. Low•Sodium Black Bean Soup

## Ingredient:

• 1 tablespoon olive oil
• 1/2 cup diced onion
• 1/2 cup diced celery
• 1/2 cup diced carrots
• 2 cloves garlic, minced
• 2 cans (15 oz each) low•sodium black beans, drained and rinsed
• 4 cups low•sodium vegetable broth
• 1 teaspoon ground cumin
• 1/2 teaspoon chili powder
• Salt and pepper to taste
• Fresh cilantro for garnish

## Instructions:

1. In a large pot, heat olive oil over medium heat.

2. Add diced onion, celery, carrots, and garlic. Cook until vegetables are tender, about 5•7 minutes.

3. Add the drained and rinsed black beans, low•sodium vegetable broth, ground cumin, and chili powder to the pot.

4. Bring the soup to a simmer and cook for about 15•20 minutes to allow the flavors to meld.

5. Season with salt and pepper to taste.

6. Use an immersion blender to partially blend the soup for a thicker consistency if desired.

7. Serve the Low•Sodium Black Bean Soup hot, garnished with fresh cilantro.

This recipe is low in sodium and phosphorus, making it suitable for a renal diet. It's important to consult with a healthcare provider or a dietitian for personalized dietary recommendations based on individual health needs.

# 40. Chicken Caesar Salad (Low Sodium Dressing)

## Ingredient:

• 4 oz grilled chicken breast, sliced
• Romaine lettuce, chopped
• 1/4 cup cherry tomatoes, halved
• 1/4 cup cucumber, sliced
• 1/4 cup shredded Parmesan cheese
• Low•sodium Caesar dressing:
  • 2 tablespoons plain Greek yogurt
  • 1 tablespoon lemon juice
  • 1 teaspoon Dijon mustard
  • 1 clove garlic, minced
  • Salt and pepper to taste

## Instructions:

1. In a large bowl, combine the chopped romaine lettuce, cherry tomatoes, cucumber, and shredded Parmesan cheese.

2. Top the salad with the sliced grilled chicken breast.

3. In a small bowl, whisk together the plain Greek yogurt, lemon juice, Dijon mustard, minced garlic, salt, and pepper to make the low•sodium Caesar dressing.

4. Drizzle the dressing over the salad and chicken.

5. Toss the salad gently to coat all ingredients with the dressing.

6. Serve the Chicken Caesar Salad with Low•Sodium Dressing as a kidney•friendly and nutritious meal option.

This recipe is low in sodium and phosphorus, making it suitable for a renal diet. It's important to consult with a healthcare provider or a dietitian for personalized dietary recommendations based on individual health needs.

# 41. Baked Salmon with Dill

## Ingredient:

• 4 oz salmon fillet
• 1 tablespoon olive oil
• 1 tablespoon fresh dill, chopped
• 1 clove garlic, minced
• 1 tablespoon lemon juice
• Salt and pepper to taste
• Lemon slices for garnish

## Instructions:

1. Preheat the oven to 375°F (190°C).

2. In a small bowl, mix together the olive oil, fresh dill, minced garlic, lemon juice, salt, and pepper.

3. Place the salmon fillet on a baking sheet lined with parchment paper.

4. Brush the dill mixture over the salmon fillet, coating it evenly.

5. Place a few lemon slices on top of the salmon.

6. Bake in the preheated oven for about 15·20 minutes or until the salmon is cooked through and flakes easily with a fork.

7. Serve the Baked Salmon with Dill hot, garnished with additional fresh dill and lemon slices.

This recipe is low in sodium and phosphorus, making it suitable for a renal diet. It's important to consult with a healthcare provider or a dietitian for personalized dietary recommendations based on individual health needs.

# 42. Grilled Chicken Breast with Herbs

## Ingredient:

• 4 boneless, skinless chicken breasts
• 2 tablespoons olive oil
• 2 cloves garlic, minced
• 1 teaspoon dried thyme
• 1 teaspoon dried rosemary
• Salt and pepper to taste
• Fresh parsley, chopped (for garnish)

## Instructions:

1. In a small bowl, mix together the olive oil, minced garlic, dried thyme, dried rosemary, salt, and pepper.

2. Rub the herb mixture over the chicken breasts, making sure they are evenly coated. Let them marinate for about 30 minutes.

3. Preheat the grill to medium•high heat.

4. Grill the chicken breasts for about 6•7 minutes per side, or until they are cooked through and reach an internal temperature of 165°F (74°C).

5. Remove the chicken from the grill and let it rest for a few minutes before serving.

6. Garnish with chopped fresh parsley before serving.

This Grilled Chicken Breast with Herbs recipe is a simple and flavorful dish that is suitable for a renal diet for seniors over 60. Enjoy the delicious herb•infused flavors of the grilled chicken!

# 43. Quinoa-Stuffed Bell Peppers

**Ingredient:**

• 4 large bell peppers, any color
• 1 cup quinoa, rinsed
• 2 cups vegetable broth
• 1 can (15 oz) black beans, drained and rinsed
• 1 can (14.5 oz) diced tomatoes, drained
• 1 cup corn kernels
• 1 small onion, diced
• 2 cloves garlic, minced
• 1 teaspoon chili powder
• 1 teaspoon cumin
• Salt and pepper to taste
• 1 cup shredded cheese (optional)
• Fresh cilantro, chopped (for garnish)

**Instructions:**

1. Preheat the oven to 375°F (190°C).

2. Cut the tops off the bell peppers and remove the seeds and membranes. Place the bell peppers in a baking dish.

3. In a saucepan, bring the vegetable broth to a boil. Add the quinoa, reduce heat to low, cover, and simmer for about 15 minutes or until the quinoa is cooked and the liquid is absorbed.

4. In a large skillet, heat some oil over medium heat. Add the diced onion and garlic, and sauté until softened.

5. Add the black beans, diced tomatoes, corn, chili powder, cumin, salt, and pepper to the skillet. Cook for a few minutes until heated through. Stir in the cooked quinoa and mix well.

6. Spoon the quinoa mixture into the bell peppers, packing it down gently. If desired, top each stuffed bell pepper with shredded cheese.

7. Cover the baking dish with foil and bake in the preheated oven for about 25•30 minutes, or until the bell peppers are tender.

8. Remove the foil and bake for an additional 5•10 minutes to melt the cheese and lightly brown the tops. Garnish with chopped fresh cilantro before serving.

# 44. Lemon Herb Tilapia

## Ingredient:

• 4 tilapia fillets
• 2 tablespoons olive oil
• 2 cloves garlic, minced
• 1 lemon, juiced and zested
• 1 teaspoon dried thyme
• 1 teaspoon dried rosemary
• Salt and pepper to taste
• Fresh parsley, chopped (for garnish)

## Instructions:

1. Preheat the oven to 400°F (200°C).

2. Place the tilapia fillets in a baking dish lightly greased with olive oil.

3. In a small bowl, mix together the olive oil, minced garlic, lemon juice, lemon zest, dried thyme, dried rosemary, salt, and pepper.

4. Pour the lemon•herb mixture over the tilapia fillets, making sure they are evenly coated.

5. Cover the baking dish with foil and bake in the preheated oven for about 15•20 minutes, or until the tilapia is cooked through and flakes easily with a fork.

6. Remove the foil and broil for an additional 2•3 minutes to lightly brown the top.

7. Garnish with chopped fresh parsley before serving.

8. Serve the Lemon Herb Tilapia hot with your favorite side dishes.

This Lemon Herb Tilapia recipe is a flavorful and kidney•friendly dish that is suitable for seniors over 60 following a renal diet. Enjoy the bright and fresh flavors of the lemon and herbs with the tender tilapia fillets!

# 45. Garlic Roasted Chicken with Vegetables

## Ingredient:

- 4 bone•in, skin•on chicken thighs
- 1 lb baby potatoes, halved
- 1 cup baby carrots
- 1 cup green beans, trimmed
- 1/2 cup cherry tomatoes
- 4 cloves garlic, minced
- 2 tablespoons olive oil
- 1 teaspoon dried thyme
- 1 teaspoon dried rosemary
- Salt and pepper to taste

## Instructions:

1. Preheat the oven to 400°F (200°C).

2. In a large bowl, combine the chicken thighs, baby potatoes, baby carrots, green beans, cherry tomatoes, minced garlic, olive oil, dried thyme, dried rosemary, salt, and pepper. Toss to coat everything evenly.

3. Arrange the chicken and vegetables in a single layer on a baking sheet lined with parchment paper.

4. Roast in the preheated oven for about 35•40 minutes or until the chicken is cooked through and the vegetables are tender, stirring halfway through cooking.

5. Once done, remove from the oven and let it rest for a few minutes before serving.

6. Serve the garlic roasted chicken with vegetables hot and enjoy!

This flavorful and nutritious Garlic Roasted Chicken with Vegetables recipe is a delicious and wholesome meal option.

# 46. Low•Sodium Beef Stir Fry

**Ingredient:**

• 1 lb lean beef (such as sirloin or flank steak), thinly sliced
• 2 tablespoons low•sodium soy sauce
• 1 tablespoon olive oil
• 2 cloves garlic, minced
• 1 teaspoon ginger, minced
• 1 red bell pepper, sliced
• 1 yellow bell pepper, sliced
• 1 cup broccoli florets
• 1 cup snap peas
• 1 small onion, sliced
• 1/4 cup low•sodium beef broth
• Salt and pepper to taste
• Cooked brown rice for serving

**Instructions:**

1. In a bowl, marinate the thinly sliced beef in low•sodium soy sauce for about 15•20 minutes.

2. Heat olive oil in a large skillet or wok over medium•high heat.

3. Add the marinated beef to the skillet and stir•fry until it is cooked to your desired level of doneness. Remove the beef from the skillet and set aside.

4. In the same skillet, add a little more oil if needed and sauté the garlic and ginger until fragrant.
5. Add the sliced bell peppers, broccoli florets, snap peas, and on
ion to the skillet. Stir•fry for a few minutes until the vegetables are slightly tender but still crisp.

6. Return the cooked beef to the skillet and pour in the low•sodium beef broth. Cook for another couple of minutes.

7. Season with salt and pepper to taste. Serve the Low•Sodium Beef Stir Fry hot over cooked brown rice.

This Low•Sodium Beef Stir Fry recipe is a kidney•friendly and flavorful dish suitable for seniors over 60 following a renal diet. Enjoy the delicious combination of beef and colorful vegetables in this stir fry!

# 47. Baked Cod with Lemon and Garlic

**Ingredient:**

• 4 cod fillets
• 2 tablespoons olive oil
• 2 cloves garlic, minced
• 1 lemon, juiced and zested
• 1 teaspoon dried oregano
• Salt and pepper to taste
• Fresh parsley, chopped (for garnish)

**Instructions:**

1. Preheat the oven to 400°F (200°C).

2. Place the cod fillets in a baking dish lightly greased with olive oil.

3. In a small bowl, mix together the olive oil, minced garlic, lemon juice, lemon zest, dried oregano, salt, and pepper.

4. Pour the lemon•garlic mixture over the cod fillets, making sure they are evenly coated.

5. Cover the baking dish with foil and bake in the preheated oven for about 15•20 minutes, or until the cod is cooked through and flakes easily with a fork.

6. Remove the foil and broil for an additional 2•3 minutes to lightly brown the top.

7. Garnish with chopped fresh parsley before serving.

8. Serve the Baked Cod with Lemon and Garlic hot with your favorite side dishes.

This Baked Cod with Lemon and Garlic recipe is simple, flavorful, and a healthy way to enjoy cod fish. Enjoy your meal!

# 48. Turkey Meatballs with Spaghetti Squash

## Ingredient:

### For the Turkey Meatballs:
• 1 lb ground turkey
• 1/4 cup breadcrumbs
• 1/4 cup grated Parmesan cheese
• 1 egg
• 2 cloves garlic, minced
• 1 teaspoon dried oregano
• Salt and pepper to taste
• 2 tablespoons olive oil

### For the Spaghetti Squash:
• 1 medium spaghetti squash
• 2 tablespoons olive oil
• Salt and pepper to taste

## Instructions:

1. Preheat the oven to 400°F (200°C).

2. Cut the spaghetti squash in half lengthwise and scoop out the seeds.

3. Brush the cut sides of the spaghetti squash with olive oil and season with salt and pepper.

4. Place the squash halves cut side down on a baking sheet and roast in the preheated oven for about 40•45 minutes, or until the squash is tender and the strands can be easily scraped with a fork.

5. While the squash is roasting, prepare the turkey meatballs. In a bowl, combine the ground turkey, breadcrumbs, Parmesan cheese, egg, minced garlic, dried oregano, salt, and pepper. Mix until well combined.

6. Shape the turkey mixture into meatballs of your desired size.

7. Heat olive oil in a skillet over medium heat. Add the turkey meatballs and cook until browned on all sides and cooked through. Once the spaghetti squash is cooked, use a fork to scrape the flesh into strands.

8. Serve the turkey meatballs over the spaghetti squash strands. Garnish with additional Parmesan cheese and fresh herbs if desired.

This Turkey Meatballs with Spaghetti Squash recipe is a healthy and delicious alternative to traditional pasta dishes. Enjoy the flavorful turkey meatballs paired with the light and nutritious spaghetti squash!

# 49. Grilled Shrimp Skewers with Veggies

## Ingredient:

• 1 lb large shrimp, peeled and deveined
• 1 red bell pepper, cut into chunks
• 1 yellow bell pepper, cut into chunks
• 1 red onion, cut into chunks
• 1 zucchini, sliced
• 1/4 cup olive oil
• 2 cloves garlic, minced
• 1 teaspoon paprika
• 1 teaspoon dried oregano
• Salt and pepper to taste
• Wooden skewers, soaked in water

## Instructions:

1. In a bowl, combine the olive oil, minced garlic, paprika, dried oregano, salt, and pepper.

2. Add the shrimp to the marinade and toss to coat. Let it marinate for about 15•20 minutes.

3. Preheat the grill to medium•high heat.

4. Thread the marinated shrimp, bell peppers, red onion, and zucchini onto the soaked wooden skewers, alternating between shrimp and veggies.

5. Brush the skewers with any remaining marinade.

6. Grill the shrimp skewers for about 2•3 minutes per side, or until the shrimp is pink and opaque.

7. Remove the skewers from the grill and serve hot.

8. You can squeeze some fresh lemon juice over the skewers before serving, if desired.

These Grilled Shrimp Skewers with Veggies are a delicious and healthy option for a meal. Enjoy the flavors of the grilled shrimp and veggies!

# 50. Chicken and Broccoli Stir Fry

## Ingredient:

• 1 lb boneless, skinless chicken breast, cut into bite•sized pieces
• 2 cups broccoli florets
• 1 red bell pepper, sliced
• 1 small onion, sliced
• 2 cloves garlic, minced
• 2 tablespoons soy sauce
• 1 tablespoon oyster sauce
• 1 teaspoon sesame oil
• 1 teaspoon cornstarch
• 1/4 cup chicken broth
• 2 tablespoons vegetable oil
• Salt and pepper to taste
• Cooked rice for serving

## Instructions:

1. In a small bowl, mix together soy sauce, oyster sauce, sesame oil, cornstarch, and chicken broth. Set aside.

2. Heat vegetable oil in a large skillet or wok over medium•high heat.

3. Add the chicken pieces to the skillet and stir•fry until they are cooked through. Remove the chicken from the skillet and set aside.

4. In the same skillet, add a little more oil if needed and sauté the garlic until fragrant.

5. Add the broccoli florets, red bell pepper, and onion to the skillet. Stir•fry for a few minutes until the vegetables are slightly tender but still crisp.

6. Return the cooked chicken to the skillet and pour the sauce mixture over the chicken and vegetables.

7. Stir well to combine and cook for another couple of minutes until the sauce thickens.

8. Season with salt and pepper to taste. Serve the Chicken and Broccoli Stir Fry hot over cooked rice.

This Chicken and Broccoli Stir Fry is a quick and flavorful dish that is perfect for a delicious and nutritious meal. Enjoy!

# 51. Herb•Crusted Pork Tenderloin

## Ingredient:

• 1 lb pork tenderloin
• 2 tablespoons Dijon mustard
• 2 cloves garlic, minced
• 1 tablespoon fresh rosemary, chopped
• 1 tablespoon fresh thyme, chopped
• 1 tablespoon fresh parsley, chopped
• Salt and pepper to taste
• 2 tablespoons olive oil

## Instructions:

1. Preheat the oven to 400°F (200°C).

2. In a small bowl, mix together the Dijon mustard, minced garlic, chopped rosemary, thyme, parsley, salt, and pepper.

3. Rub the pork tenderloin with the herb mixture, making sure to coat it evenly.

4. Heat olive oil in an oven•safe skillet over medium•high heat.

5. Sear the pork tenderloin on all sides until browned, about 2•3 minutes per side.

6. Transfer the skillet to the preheated oven and roast the pork tenderloin for about 20•25 minutes, or until the internal temperature reaches 145°F (63°C).

7. Remove the pork tenderloin from the oven and let it rest for a few minutes before slicing.

8. Slice the Herb•Crusted Pork Tenderloin and serve hot with your favorite side dishes.

This Herb•Crusted Pork Tenderloin recipe is a flavorful and elegant dish that is perfect for a special meal. Enjoy the delicious herb•infused flavors of the pork tenderloin!

# 52. Veggie and Tofu Stir Fry

**Ingredient:**

• 14 oz firm tofu, drained and cubed
• 2 tablespoons soy sauce
• 1 tablespoon sesame oil
• 1 tablespoon cornstarch
• 2 tablespoons vegetable oil
• 2 cloves garlic, minced
• 1 teaspoon ginger, minced
• 1 red bell pepper, sliced
• 1 yellow bell pepper, sliced
• 1 cup broccoli florets
• 1 cup snap peas
• 1 medium carrot, sliced
• 1/4 cup low•sodium vegetable broth
• Salt and pepper to taste
• Cooked rice or noodles for serving

**Instructions:**

1. In a bowl, combine the cubed tofu with soy sauce, sesame oil, and cornstarch. Toss gently to coat the tofu evenly and set aside.

2. Heat vegetable oil in a large skillet or wok over medium•high heat.

3. Add the marinated tofu to the skillet and cook until golden brown o all sides. Remove the tofu from the skillet and set aside.

4. In the same skillet, add a little more oil if needed and sauté the garlic and ginger until fragrant.

5. Add the sliced bell peppers, broccoli, snap peas, and carrot to the skillet. Stir•fry for a few minutes until the vegetables are slightly tender but still crisp.

6. Pour in the vegetable broth and cook for another couple of minutes.

7. Return the cooked tofu to the skillet and toss everything together. Season with salt and pepper to taste. Serve the Veggie and Tofu Stir Fry over cooked rice or noodles.

This Veggie and Tofu Stir Fry is a healthy and delicious dish packed with protein and colorful vegetables. Enjoy!

# 53. Spaghetti with Garlic and Olive Oil

## Ingredient:

• 8 oz whole wheat spaghetti
• 4 cloves garlic, thinly sliced
• 1/4 cup olive oil
• Red pepper flakes (optional)
• Salt and pepper to taste
• Fresh parsley, chopped (for garnish)

## Instructions:

1. Cook the whole wheat spaghetti according to the package instructions until al dente. Drain and set aside.

2. In a large skillet, heat the olive oil over medium heat.

3. Add the thinly sliced garlic to the skillet and sauté until fragrant and lightly golden, about 1•2 minutes. Be careful not to burn the garlic.

4. If desired, add a pinch of red pepper flakes for a bit of heat.

5. Add the cooked spaghetti to the skillet and toss to coat the pasta with the garlic•infused olive oil.

6. Season with salt and pepper to taste.

7. Serve the Spaghetti with Garlic and Olive Oil hot, garnished with chopped fresh parsley.

This simple and flavorful Spaghetti with Garlic and Olive Oil recipe is a kidney•friendly option for seniors over 60 following a renal diet. Enjoy the classic combination of garlic and olive oil with whole wheat spaghetti for a delicious and satisfying meal!

# 54. Baked Chicken Thighs with Rosemary

**Ingredient:**

• 4 bone•in, skin•on chicken thighs
• 2 tablespoons olive oil
• 2 cloves garlic, minced
• 1 tablespoon fresh rosemary, chopped
• 1 lemon, juiced and zested
• Salt and pepper to taste

**Instructions**:

1. Preheat the oven to 400°F (200°C).

2. In a small bowl, mix together the olive oil, minced garlic, chopped rosemary, lemon juice, lemon zest, salt, and pepper.

3. Rub the mixture over the chicken thighs, making sure they are evenly coated.

4. Place the chicken thighs in a baking dish.

5. Bake in the preheated oven for about 35•40 minutes, or until the chicken is cooked through and the skin is crispy.

6. Remove from the oven and let it rest for a few minutes before serving.

7. Garnish with additional fresh rosemary before serving.

This Baked Chicken Thighs with Rosemary recipe is a flavorful and kidney•friendly dish suitable for seniors over 60 following a renal diet. Enjoy the aromatic rosemary•infused flavors of the baked chicken thighs!

# 55. Low•Sodium Chili with Ground Turkey

**Ingredient:**

• 1 lb lean ground turkey
• 1 onion, diced
• 2 cloves garlic, minced
• 1 red bell pepper, diced
• 1 can (15 oz) low•sodium kidney beans, drained and rinsed
• 1 can (15 oz) low•sodium diced tomatoes
• 1 cup low•sodium chicken broth
• 1 tablespoon chili powder
• 1 teaspoon cumin
• 1/2 teaspoon paprika
• Salt and pepper to taste
• Optional toppings: chopped fresh cilantro, low•sodium shredded cheese, low•fat sour cream

**Instructions:**

1. In a large pot or Dutch oven, cook the ground turkey over medium heat until browned.

2. Add the diced onion, minced garlic, and diced red bell pepper to the pot. Cook until the vegetables are softened.

3. Stir in the low•sodium kidney beans, low•sodium diced tomatoes, and low•sodium chicken broth.

4. Add the chili powder, cumin, paprika, salt, and pepper. Stir to combine.

5. Bring the chili to a simmer, then reduce the heat to low. Cover and let it simmer for about 30•40 minutes, stirring occasionally.

6. Adjust the seasoning with salt and pepper if needed.

7. Serve the Low•Sodium Chili with Ground Turkey hot, garnished with optional toppings like chopped fresh cilantro, low•sodium shredded cheese, or low•fat sour cream.

This Low•Sodium Chili with Ground Turkey recipe is a kidney•friendly and flavorful dish suitable for seniors over 60 following a renal diet. Enjoy the hearty and comforting flavors of this low•sodium chili!

# 56. Stuffed Zucchini Boats

**Ingredient:**

• 4 medium zucchinis
• 1/2 lb lean ground turkey
• 1 small onion, diced
• 1 bell pepper, diced
• 2 cloves garlic, minced
• 1 can (14.5 oz) low•sodium diced tomatoes
• 1/2 cup low•sodium chicken broth
• 1 teaspoon dried oregano
• 1 teaspoon dried basil
• Salt and pepper to taste
• 1/4 cup grated Parmesan cheese
• Fresh parsley, chopped (for garnish)

**Instructions:**
1. Preheat the oven to 375°F (190°C).

2. Cut the zucchinis in half lengthwise and scoop out the seeds to create a hollow center for the boats.

3. In a skillet, cook the ground turkey over medium heat until browned. Add the diced onion, bell pepper, and garlic, and cook until the vegetables are softened.

4. Stir in the low•sodium diced tomatoes, low•sodium chicken broth, dried oregano, dried basil, salt, and pepper. Simmer for a few minutes.

5. Fill each zucchini boat with the turkey and vegetable mixture.

6. Place the stuffed zucchini boats in a baking dish and cover with foil.

7. Bake in the preheated oven for about 25•30 minutes, or until the zucchinis are tender.

8. Remove the foil, sprinkle the grated Parmesan cheese over the zucchini boats, and bake for an additional 5•10 minutes until the cheese is melted and bubbly. Garnish with chopped fresh parsley before serving.

These Stuffed Zucchini Boats are a kidney•friendly and nutritious dish suitable for seniors over 60 following a renal diet. Enjoy the flavorful and wholesome combination of zucchinis, ground turkey, and vegetables in this satisfying meal!

# 57. Herb•Roasted Turkey Breast

**Ingredient:**

• 2 lbs turkey breast, bone•in and skinless
• 2 tablespoons olive oil
• 2 cloves garlic, minced
• 1 tablespoon fresh rosemary, chopped
• 1 tablespoon fresh thyme, chopped
• 1 tablespoon fresh parsley, chopped
• Salt and pepper to taste

**Instructions**:

1. Preheat the oven to 375°F (190°C).

2. In a small bowl, mix together the olive oil, minced garlic, chopped rosemary, thyme, parsley, salt, and pepper.

3. Rub the herb mixture over the turkey breast, making sure it is evenly coated.

4. Place the turkey breast in a roasting pan.

5. Roast in the preheated oven for about 1 to 1.5 hours, or until the internal temperature reaches 165°F (74°C) and the turkey is cooked through.

6. Baste the turkey breast with the pan juices occasionally during cooking.

7. Remove the turkey breast from the oven and let it rest for a few minutes before slicing.

8. Slice the Herb•Roasted Turkey Breast and serve hot.

This Herb•Roasted Turkey Breast recipe is a kidney•friendly and flavorful dish suitable for seniors over 60 following a renal diet. Enjoy the aromatic herb•infused flavors of the roasted turkey breast!

# 58. Grilled Lamb Chops with Mint

**Ingredient:**

• 4 lamb chops
• 2 tablespoons olive oil
• 2 cloves garlic, minced
• 1 tablespoon fresh mint, chopped
• 1 teaspoon dried oregano
• Salt and pepper to taste
• Lemon wedges (for serving)

**Instructions**:

1. In a bowl, mix together the olive oil, minced garlic, chopped mint, dried oregano, salt, and pepper.

2. Rub the mixture over the lamb chops, making sure they are evenly coated. Let them marinate for about 30 minutes.

3. Preheat the grill to medium•high heat.

4. Grill the lamb chops for about 3•4 minutes per side for medium•rare, or longer to your desired level of doneness.

5. Remove the lamb chops from the grill and let them rest for a few minutes before serving.

6. Serve the Grilled Lamb Chops with Mint hot, garnished with additional fresh mint and lemon wedges on the side.

This Grilled Lamb Chops with Mint recipe is a flavorful and elegant dish that is perfect for a special meal. Enjoy the combination of tender lamb chops with the refreshing taste of mint!

# 59. Chicken Marsala (Low Sodium)

**Ingredient:**

• 4 boneless, skinless chicken breasts
• 1/4 cup all•purpose flour
• 1/2 teaspoon garlic powder
• 1/2 teaspoon onion powder
• 1/2 teaspoon dried thyme
• 1/2 teaspoon dried oregano
• Salt and pepper to taste
• 2 tablespoons olive oil
• 1 cup low•sodium chicken broth
• 1 cup Marsala wine
• 8 oz mushrooms, sliced
• Fresh parsley, chopped (for garnish)

**Instructions**:

1. In a shallow dish, mix together the flour, garlic powder, onion powder, dried thyme, dried oregano, salt, and pepper.

2. Dredge the chicken breasts in the seasoned flour mixture, shaking off any excess. In a large skillet, heat the olive oil over medium•high heat.

4. Add the chicken breasts to the skillet and cook until browned on both sides and cooked through. Remove the chicken from the skillet and set aside.

5. In the same skillet, add the sliced mushrooms and sauté until they are tender.

6. Pour in the low•sodium chicken broth and Marsala wine, scraping up any browned bits from the bottom of the skillet.

7. Bring the sauce to a simmer and cook for a few minutes until it slightly thickens.

8. Return the chicken breasts to the skillet and simmer in the sauce for a couple of minutes to heat through.

9. Season with additional salt and pepper if needed. Garnish with chopped fresh parsley before serving.

This Low•Sodium Chicken Marsala recipe is a kidney•friendly version of the classic dish, suitable for seniors over 60 following a renal diet. Enjoy the rich flavors of the Marsala wine sauce with tender chicken and mushrooms!

# 60. Cauliflower Fried Rice

**Ingredient:**

• 1 head of cauliflower
• 2 tablespoons olive oil
• 2 cloves garlic, minced
• 1 small onion, diced
• 1 carrot, diced
• 1/2 cup frozen peas
• 2 eggs, beaten
• 2 tablespoons low•sodium soy sauce
• Salt and pepper to taste
• Green onions, chopped (for garnish)

**Instructions:**

1. Cut the cauliflower into florets and pulse in a food processor until it resembles rice grains.

2. In a large skillet or wok, heat olive oil over medium heat.

3. Add the minced garlic and diced onion to the skillet and sauté until softened.

4. Add the diced carrot and frozen peas to the skillet and cook until the vegetables are tender.

5. Push the vegetables to one side of the skillet and pour the beaten eggs into the other side. Scramble the eggs until cooked through.

6. Mix the scrambled eggs with the vegetables in the skillet.

7. Add the riced cauliflower to the skillet and stir to combine with the vegetables and eggs.

8. Drizzle the low•sodium soy sauce over the cauliflower fried rice and mix well.

9. Season with salt and pepper to taste. Cook for a few more minutes until the cauliflower is tender but not mushy. Garnish with chopped green onions before serving.

This Cauliflower Fried Rice recipe is a kidney•friendly and low•carb alternative to traditional fried rice, suitable for seniors over 60 following a renal diet. Enjoy the nutritious and flavorful cauliflower rice dish!

# 61. Apple Slices with Peanut Butter

**Ingredient:**

• 1 medium apple, sliced
• 2 tablespoons unsalted peanut butter

**Instructions:**

1. Wash and slice the apple into thin wedges or rounds.

2. Serve the apple slices with a side of unsalted peanut butter for dipping.

3. Enjoy the combination of the crisp apple slices with the creamy peanut butter as a nutritious and satisfying snack.

This Apple Slices with Peanut Butter recipe is a healthy and kidney•friendly option for seniors over 60 following a renal diet. It provides a balance of fiber, vitamins, and protein for a tasty and easy snack.

# 62. Carrot Sticks with Hummus

**Ingredient:**

• 2 large carrots, peeled and cut into sticks
• 1 can (15 oz) of low•sodium chickpeas, drained and rinsed
• 2 tablespoons of tahini
• 2 tablespoons of lemon juice
• 1 clove of garlic, minced
• 1/4 teaspoon of cumin
• Salt and pepper to taste
• Water (as needed for desired consistency)

**Instructions:**

1. Steam or blanch the carrot sticks until they are tender but still slightly crisp. Let them cool before serving.

2. In a food processor, combine the chickpeas, tahini, lemon juice, garlic, cumin, salt, and pepper. Blend until smooth, adding water as needed to reach your desired consistency.

3. Transfer the hummus to a serving bowl and serve with the carrot sticks on the side.

This snack is not only delicious but also provides a good source of fiber, protein, and essential nutrients for seniors following a renal diet. Enjoy!

# 63. Unsalted Almonds

**Ingredient:**

• Unsalted almonds

**Instructions:**

1. Portion out a serving of unsalted almonds. A typical serving size is about 1 ounce, which is roughly a handful of almonds.

2. Enjoy the almonds as a snack on their own, or you can mix them with other unsalted nuts or seeds for variety.

3. Remember to chew the almonds thoroughly to aid digestion.

Almonds are a good source of healthy fats, protein, fiber, and essential nutrients like vitamin E and magnesium. They can be a satisfying and kidney•friendly snack for individuals following a renal diet.

# 64. Rice Cakes with Cottage Cheese

**Ingredient:**

• Rice cakes
• Cottage cheese
• Optional toppings: sliced fruits (such as berries or bananas), a drizzle of honey, or a sprinkle of cinnamon

**Instructions:**

1. Spread a layer of cottage cheese on top of a rice cake.

2. Add your choice of toppings, such as sliced fruits, a drizzle of honey, or a sprinkle of cinnamon.

3. Enjoy your rice cake with cottage cheese as a light and tasty snack.

This snack provides a good balance of carbohydrates, protein, and healthy fats. It can be a convenient option for a quick and nutritious bite, especially for those following a renal diet. Feel free to customize the toppings to suit your taste preferences.

# 65. Greek Yogurt with Honey

**Ingredient:**

• 1 cup Greek yogurt (low•fat or non•fat)
• 1•2 tablespoons honey
• Fresh berries or sliced fruit (optional)
• Chopped nuts (optional)

**Instructions:**

1. Spoon the Greek yogurt into a serving bowl.

2. Drizzle the honey over the yogurt.

3. If desired, top with fresh berries or sliced fruit for added flavor and nutrients.

4. Optionally, sprinkle chopped nuts on top for some crunch and extra protein. Serve the Greek Yogurt with Honey as a nutritious and satisfying snack or dessert.

This Greek Yogurt with Honey recipe is a kidney•friendly and delicious option for seniors over 60 following a renal diet. Enjoy the creamy yogurt paired with the natural sweetness of honey for a simple and wholesome treat.

# 66. Celery Sticks with Low•Sodium Cheese

**Ingredient:**

• Celery sticks, washed and cut into manageable lengths
• Low•sodium cheese, such as Swiss or mozzarella, sliced or cubed

**Instructions:**

1. Take a celery stick and fill the center crevice with slices or cubes of low•sodium cheese.

2. Repeat with the remaining celery sticks and cheese.

3. Enjoy the celery sticks with low•sodium cheese as a crunchy and satisfying snack.

This snack provides a good balance of fiber, protein, and essential nutrients while keeping sodium levels in check, which is important for individuals following a renal diet. Feel free to adjust the portion sizes to meet your dietary needs and preferences.

# 67. Blueberries and Almonds Mix

**Ingredient:**

• Fresh blueberries
• Unsalted almonds

**Instructions:**

1. Wash the blueberries and portion them out into a bowl.

2. Measure out a serving of unsalted almonds.

3. Combine the blueberries and almonds in a bowl to create a tasty and kidney•friendly snack mix.

4. Enjoy the mix as a healthy snack option.

Blueberries are rich in antioxidants and fiber, while almonds provide healthy fats, protein, and essential nutrients. This snack mix offers a good balance of nutrients and can be a satisfying option for seniors following a renal diet. Feel free to adjust the portion sizes to suit your preferences.

# 68. Unsweetened Applesauce

**Ingredient:**

• 6•8 apples (such as Granny Smith or Fuji), peeled, cored, and sliced
• Water
• Cinnamon (optional)

**Instructions:**

1. In a large pot, combine the sliced apples with enough water to cover the bottom of the pot.

2. Bring the water to a simmer over medium heat.

3. Cover the pot and cook the apples, stirring occasionally, until they are soft and easily mashed with a fork.

4. Remove the pot from the heat and let the apples cool slightly.

5. Mash the cooked apples with a potato masher or blend them in a food processor until you reach your desired consistency.

6. If desired, add a sprinkle of cinnamon for flavor.

7. Let the unsweetened applesauce cool completely before serving or storing in the refrigerator.

This Unsweetened Applesauce recipe is a kidney•friendly and nutritious option for seniors over 60 following a renal diet. Enjoy the natural sweetness and comforting taste of homemade applesauce without added sugars.

# 69. Low•Sodium Popcorn

**Ingredient:**

• Plain popcorn kernels
• Olive oil or canola oil
• Salt•free seasoning blend (optional)

**Instructions**:
1. Heat a large pot over medium heat and add a small amount of olive oil or canola oil.

2. Add the popcorn kernels to the pot, covering the bottom in a single layer. Cover the pot with a lid and shake it gently to coat the kernels with oil.

3. Allow the popcorn to pop, shaking the pot occasionally to prevent burning. Once the popping slows down, remove the pot from the heat. Transfer the popcorn to a bowl and sprinkle with a salt•free seasoning blend if desired.

This low•sodium popcorn recipe provides a crunchy and satisfying snack option for seniors following a renal diet. Popcorn is a whole grain that is high in fiber and can be a healthier alternative to traditional salty snacks. Enjoy your low•sodium popcorn as a guilt•free treat!

# 70. Sliced Bell Peppers with Guacamole

**Ingredient:**

• Bell peppers (choose a variety of colors for a vibrant presentation)
• Ripe avocados
• Lime juice
• Salt and pepper to taste
• Optional toppings: diced tomatoes, chopped cilantro, minced garlic, or a sprinkle of chili powder

**Instructions:**
1. Wash and slice the bell peppers into strips or wedges.

2. In a bowl, mash the ripe avocados with lime juice, salt, and pepper to make guacamole. You can also add optional toppings like diced tomatoes, chopped cilantro, minced garlic, or a sprinkle of chili powder for extra flavor. Serve the sliced bell peppers with the guacamole for dipping.

This snack is rich in vitamins, minerals, healthy fats, and fiber, making it a nutritious choice for seniors over 60 following a renal diet. The combination of bell peppers and guacamole provides a satisfying and kidney•friendly snack option. Enjoy!

# 71. Strawberries with Whipped Cream

**Ingredient:**

• Fresh strawberries, washed and hulled
• Whipped cream (you can use a light or sugar•free version for a healthier option)

**Instructions:**
1. Place the fresh strawberries in a bowl or on a plate.

2. Top the strawberries with a dollop of whipped cream.

3. You can garnish with a mint leaf or a sprinkle of cinnamon for added flavor, if desired.

4. Enjoy the strawberries with whipped cream as a sweet and refreshing treat.

This dessert provides a balance of natural sweetness from the strawberries and the creamy texture of the whipped cream. It can be a satisfying option for seniors over 60 following a renal diet. Remember to enjoy this treat in moderation as part of a balanced diet.

# 72. Cherry Tomatoes with Basil and Olive Oil

**Ingredient:**

• 1 pint cherry tomatoes, halved
• 2 tablespoons extra•virgin olive oil
• 2 tablespoons fresh basil, chopped
• Salt and pepper to taste

**Instructions:**
1. In a bowl, combine the halved cherry tomatoes, extra•virgin olive oil, and chopped fresh basil.

2. Toss gently to coat the cherry tomatoes evenly with the olive oil and basil. Season with salt and pepper to taste. Let the flavors meld together for a few minutes before serving.

3. Serve the Cherry Tomatoes with Basil and Olive Oil as a refreshing and light side dish.

This Cherry Tomatoes with Basil and Olive Oil recipe is a flavorful and kidney•friendly option for seniors over 60 following a renal diet. Enjoy the vibrant colors and fresh flavors of this simple dish!

# 73. Pear Slices with Ricotta

**Ingredient:**

• Ripe pears, washed and sliced
• Ricotta cheese
• Optional: a drizzle of honey or a sprinkle of cinnamon for added sweetness

**Instructions:**

1. Wash and slice the pears into thin wedges or slices.

2. Spread a layer of ricotta cheese on a plate or serving dish.

3. Arrange the pear slices on top of the ricotta.

4. Drizzle a little honey or sprinkle cinnamon over the pear slices for extra flavor, if desired. Enjoy the pear slices with ricotta as a tasty and kidney•friendly snack.

Pears are a good source of fiber and vitamins, while ricotta cheese provides protein and calcium. This snack combination offers a balance of nutrients and flavors that can be enjoyed as a light and satisfying treat. Feel free to adjust the portion sizes to suit your preferences.

# 74. Air•Popped Popcorn

**Ingredient:**

• Popcorn kernels
• Optional: a sprinkle of salt or other seasonings of your choice (such as nutritional yeast, garlic powder, or chili powder)

**Instructions:**

1. Place a handful of popcorn kernels in an air popper.

2. Turn on the air popper and let it pop the kernels until they are all popped.

3. Transfer the air•popped popcorn to a bowl.

4. If desired, sprinkle a little salt or other seasonings over the popcorn for added flavor.

5. Toss the popcorn to distribute the seasonings evenly.

6. Enjoy the air•popped popcorn as a light and crunchy snack.

Air•popped popcorn is a whole grain snack that is low in calories and provides fiber. It can be a satisfying option for seniors following a renal diet. Feel free to customize the seasonings to suit your taste preferences and enjoy this guilt•free snack!

# 75. Cucumber Slices with Dill Dip

## Ingredient:

- Cucumber, washed and sliced
- Plain Greek yogurt
- Fresh dill, chopped
- Lemon juice
- Garlic powder
- Salt and pepper to taste

## Instructions:

1. In a small bowl, mix together plain Greek yogurt, chopped fresh dill, a splash of lemon juice, a pinch of garlic powder, salt, and pepper.

2. Stir the ingredients until well combined to create the dill dip.

3. Arrange the cucumber slices on a plate or platter. Serve the cucumber slices with the dill dip on the side for dipping.

This snack is low in sodium and provides a good source of hydration, vitamins, and minerals. It's a light and kidney•friendly option for seniors over 60. The combination of cool cucumber and flavorful dill dip makes for a tasty and satisfying snack. Enjoy!

# 76. Baked Kale Chips

**Ingredient:**

• Fresh kale leaves, washed and dried
• Olive oil
• Salt and pepper, or other seasonings of your choice (such as garlic powder, paprika, or nutritional yeast)

**Instructions:**

1. Preheat the oven to 300°F (150°C).

2. Remove the tough stems from the kale leaves and tear the leaves into bite•sized pieces.

3. In a bowl, toss the kale pieces with a drizzle of olive oil until evenly coated.

4. Spread the kale pieces in a single layer on a baking sheet lined with parchment paper.

5. Season the kale with salt, pepper, or other seasonings of your choice.

6. Bake in the preheated oven for about 10•15 minutes, or until the kale is crispy but not burnt. Remove from the oven and let the kale chips cool before serving.

Baked kale chips are a crunchy and flavorful snack that provides fiber, vitamins, and minerals. They are a healthy alternative to traditional potato chips and can be a satisfying option for seniors following a renal diet. Enjoy the crispy goodness of homemade baked kale chips!

# 77. Watermelon Cubes

## Ingredient:

• Fresh watermelon
• Optional: a sprinkle of salt or a squeeze of lime juice for added flavor

## Instructions:

1. Wash the watermelon and cut it into cubes, removing any seeds if necessary.

2. Place the watermelon cubes in a bowl or on a plate.

3. If desired, you can sprinkle a little salt over the watermelon cubes for a sweet and salty contrast, or squeeze some fresh lime juice for a tangy kick.

4. Enjoy the watermelon cubes as a light and hydrating snack.

Watermelon is a good source of hydration, vitamins, and antioxidants. It's a kidney•friendly fruit that can be enjoyed by seniors over 60 as a healthy snack option. Feel free to adjust the portion sizes to suit your preferences and enjoy the refreshing taste of watermelon cubes.

# 78. Low•Sodium Crackers with Cheese

## Ingredient:

• Low•sodium whole grain crackers
• Low•sodium cheese (such as Swiss or mozzarella)
• Fresh herbs (such as parsley or chives) for garnish

## Instructions:

1. Preheat the oven to 350°F (180°C).

2. Place the low•sodium whole grain crackers on a baking sheet lined with parchment paper. Thinly slice the low•sodium cheese and place a slice on each cracker.

3. Bake in the preheated oven for about 5•7 minutes, or until the cheese is melted. Remove from the oven and let cool slightly. Garnish with fresh herbs before serving.

These low•sodium crackers with cheese are a tasty and kidney•friendly snack option for seniors over 60 following a renal diet. The whole grain crackers provide fiber, while the low•sodium cheese adds protein and calcium. Enjoy these crackers as a satisfying and nutritious snack!

# 79. Rice Pudding

**Ingredient:**

• 1/2 cup white rice
• 4 cups milk
• 1/3 cup sugar
• 1/4 tsp salt
• 1 tsp vanilla extract
• 1/2 tsp ground cinnamon
• Optional toppings: raisins, nuts, or a sprinkle of cinnamon

**Instructions**:
1. In a medium saucepan, combine the rice, milk, sugar, and salt.

2. Bring the mixture to a boil over medium heat, stirring occasionally.

3. Reduce the heat to low and simmer, stirring frequently, for about 20•25 minutes or until the rice is cooked and the mixture has thickened.

4. Remove the saucepan from the heat and stir in the vanilla extract.

5. Let the rice pudding cool slightly before serving. Sprinkle ground cinnamon on top and add any optional toppings if desired.

Enjoy this creamy and comforting rice pudding warm or chilled. It's a classic dessert that is sure to be a hit with family and friends!

# 80. Dried Apricots (Unsulfured)

**Ingredient:**

- 2 cups dried unsulfured apricots
- 1 cup almonds
- 1/2 cup shredded coconut
- 1/4 cup honey
- 1/4 cup coconut oil
- 1 tsp vanilla extract
- Pinch of salt

**Instructions**:

1. In a food processor, pulse the almonds until finely chopped.

2. Add the dried apricots, shredded coconut, honey, coconut oil, vanilla extract, and salt to the food processor. Pulse until the mixture comes together and forms a sticky dough.

3. Line a baking dish with parchment paper and press the mixture evenly into the dish.

4. Refrigerate for at least 1 hour to set.

5. Once set, cut into bars and enjoy!

These dried apricot bars are a delicious and healthy snack that you can enjoy on the go. Feel free to customize the recipe by adding in other nuts or seeds for extra crunch!

# 81. Lemon Sorbet

## Ingredient:

- 1 cup water
- 1 cup sugar
- 1 cup freshly squeezed lemon juice (about 4·6 lemons)
- Zest of 1 lemon

## Instructions:

1. In a small saucepan, combine the water and sugar. Heat over medium heat, stirring occasionally, until the sugar is completely dissolved to create a simple syrup. Remove from heat and let it cool.

2. In a mixing bowl, combine the lemon juice and lemon zest.

3. Once the simple syrup has cooled, mix it into the lemon juice and zest mixture.

4. Pour the mixture into a shallow dish or a container suitable for freezing.

5. Place the dish in the freezer and let it freeze for about 2·3 hours.

6. Every 30 minutes, take the dish out of the freezer and stir the mixture with a fork to break up any ice crystals. Repeat this process until the sorbet is frozen and has a smooth texture.

7. Once the sorbet is ready, scoop it into serving dishes and garnish with a slice of lemon or mint leaves if desired.

This homemade Lemon Sorbet is a light and tangy dessert that is perfect for cooling down on a hot day. Enjoy the bright and refreshing flavors of lemon in this delightful frozen treat!

# 82. Fresh Fruit Salad

**Ingredient:**

• Assorted fresh fruits (such as strawberries, blueberries, kiwi, pineapple, grapes, and oranges)
• Fresh mint leaves (optional, for garnish)
• Honey or a splash of citrus juice (optional, for added sweetness)

**Instructions:**

1. Wash, peel, and chop the fruits into bite•sized pieces.

2. Combine the assorted fruits in a large bowl.

3. If desired, drizzle a little honey or a splash of citrus juice over the fruit salad for added sweetness.

4. Gently toss the fruits to mix them together.

5. Garnish with fresh mint leaves for a pop of color and flavor.

6. Serve the fresh fruit salad chilled and enjoy!

This fruit salad is a nutritious and kidney•friendly option for seniors over 60. It's packed with vitamins, minerals, and antioxidants from a variety of fresh fruits. Feel free to customize the fruit selection based on your preferences and what's in season. Enjoy this refreshing and healthy snack or dessert!

# 83. Rice Krispie Treats

**Ingredient:**

• 6 cups crispy rice cereal (such as Rice Krispies)
• 4 cups mini marshmallows
• 3 tablespoons unsalted butter

**Instructions:**

1. Grease a 9x13•inch baking dish with butter or cooking spray.

2. In a large saucepan, melt the butter over low heat.

3. Add the mini marshmallows to the melted butter and stir continuously until the marshmallows are completely melted and smooth.

4. Remove the saucepan from the heat and quickly stir in the crispy rice cereal until it is evenly coated with the marshmallow mixture.

5. Transfer the mixture to the prepared baking dish and press it down evenly with a spatula or your hands.

6. Let the Rice Krispie treats cool and set for about 30 minutes before cutting into squares.

These Rice Krispie Treats are a simple and delicious snack that is loved by both kids and adults. Enjoy the crispy, chewy goodness of these classic treats!

# 84. Vanilla Pudding

**Ingredient:**

- 2/3 cup granulated sugar
- 1/4 cup cornstarch
- 1/4 teaspoon salt
- 3 cups whole milk
- 4 large egg yolks
- 2 tablespoons unsalted butter
- 2 teaspoons vanilla extract

**Instructions:**

1. In a medium saucepan, whisk together the sugar, cornstarch, and salt.

2. In a separate bowl, whisk together the milk and egg yolks until well combined.

3. Gradually whisk the milk mixture into the sugar mixture in the saucepan.

4. Cook the mixture over medium heat, stirring constantly, until it thickens and comes to a boil. This should take about 8•10 minutes.

5. Remove the saucepan from the heat and stir in the butter and vanilla extract until the butter is melted and the mixture is smooth.

6. Pour the pudding into individual serving dishes or a large bowl.

7. Cover the pudding with plastic wrap, making sure the wrap touches the surface of the pudding to prevent a skin from forming.

8. Refrigerate the pudding for at least 2 hours, or until chilled and set.

This homemade Vanilla Pudding is creamy, smooth, and bursting with vanilla flavor. Enjoy it on its own or use it as a delicious filling for cakes, pies, or parfaits. It's a classic dessert that is sure to be a hit with family and friends!

# 85. Apple Crisp (Low Sugar)

**Ingredient:**

• 4 cups peeled and sliced apples
• 1/4 cup unsweetened applesauce
• 1/4 cup rolled oats
• 1/4 cup almond flour
• 1/4 cup chopped walnuts
• 1/2 tsp cinnamon
• 1/4 tsp nutmeg
• 1/4 tsp salt
• 1 tbsp honey or maple syrup (optional)

**Instructions:**

1. Preheat the oven to 350°F (180°C).

2. In a bowl, combine the sliced apples and unsweetened applesauce. Spread the mixture in a baking dish.

3. In another bowl, mix the rolled oats, almond flour, chopped walnuts, cinnamon, nutmeg, and salt. If desired, you can add a small amount of honey or maple syrup for sweetness.

4. Sprinkle the oat mixture evenly over the apples in the baking dish.

5. Bake in the preheated oven for about 30•35 minutes, or until the topping is golden brown and the apples are tender.

6. Allow the apple crisp to cool slightly before serving.

This Low•Sugar Apple Crisp is a kidney•friendly dessert option for seniors over 60 following a renal diet. The use of unsweetened applesauce and a small amount of honey or maple syrup keeps the sugar content low while still providing a delicious and comforting treat. Enjoy this apple crisp warm with a dollop of low•sugar whipped cream or a scoop of vanilla ice cream if desired.

# 86. Baked Apples with Cinnamon

## Ingredient:

• 4 medium•sized apples (such as Granny Smith or Honeycrisp)
• 2 tablespoons unsalted butter, melted
• 2 tablespoons brown sugar
• 1 teaspoon ground cinnamon
• 1/4 cup chopped nuts (such as walnuts or pecans), optional
• Vanilla ice cream or whipped cream for serving, optional

## Instructions:

1. Preheat the oven to 375°F (190°C).

2. Core the apples using an apple corer or a knife, leaving the bottom intact to create a well for the filling.

3. In a small bowl, mix together the melted butter, brown sugar, and cinnamon.

4. Place the cored apples in a baking dish and fill each apple with the buttery cinnamon mixture.

5. If using chopped nuts, sprinkle them over the top of the apples.

6. Cover the baking dish with foil and bake in the preheated oven for about 25•30 minutes, or until the apples are tender.

7. Remove the foil and bake for an additional 5•10 minutes to allow the tops to caramelize slightly.

8. Serve the baked apples warm, optionally topped with a scoop of vanilla ice cream or a dollop of whipped cream.

These Baked Apples with Cinnamon are a comforting and flavorful dessert that is perfect for fall or any time you're craving a sweet treat. Enjoy the warm, tender apples with a hint of cinnamon and a crunchy nut topping for a delightful dessert experience!

# 87. Peach Cobbler (Low Sugar)

**Ingredient:**

• 4 cups sliced fresh peaches (or canned peaches in juice, drained)
• 1/4 cup sugar (or sweetener of your choice)
• 1/2 teaspoon cinnamon
• 1/4 teaspoon nutmeg
• 1 cup all•purpose flour
• 1/4 cup almond flour
• 1/4 cup rolled oats
• 1/4 cup unsweetened applesauce
• 1/4 cup unsalted butter, melted
• 1/4 cup milk (or almond milk)
• 1 teaspoon baking powder
• 1/4 teaspoon salt

**Instructions**:
1. Preheat the oven to 375°F (190°C).

2. In a bowl, combine the sliced peaches, sugar, cinnamon, and nutmeg. Mix well and spread the mixture in a baking dish.

3. In another bowl, mix the all•purpose flour, almond flour, rolled oats, baking powder, and salt.

4. Add the unsweetened applesauce, melted butter, and milk to the flour mixture. Stir until just combined.

5. Drop spoonfuls of the batter over the peaches in the baking dish.

6. Bake in the preheated oven for about 30•35 minutes, or until the topping is golden brown and the peaches are bubbly.

7. Allow the peach cobbler to cool slightly before serving.

This Low•Sugar Peach Cobbler is a delightful dessert that highlights the natural sweetness of fresh peaches without adding too much sugar. Enjoy this warm cobbler on its own or with a dollop of low•sugar whipped cream or a scoop of vanilla ice cream for a special treat!

# 88. Strawberry Shortcake

**Ingredient:**

• 1 quart fresh strawberries, hulled and sliced
• 1/4 cup sugar
• 2 cups all•purpose flour
• 1/4 cup sugar
• 1 tablespoon baking powder
• 1/2 teaspoon salt
• 1/2 cup cold unsalted butter, cut into small pieces
• 2/3 cup milk
• Whipped cream for topping

**Instructions:**

1. In a bowl, mix the sliced strawberries with 1/4 cup of sugar. Let them sit for about 30 minutes to allow the strawberries to release their juices.

2. Preheat the oven to 425°F (220°C).

3. In a large bowl, whisk together the flour, 1/4 cup sugar, baking powder, and salt.

4. Cut in the cold butter using a pastry cutter or your fingers until the mixture resembles coarse crumbs.

5. Stir in the milk until just combined to form a dough.

6. Turn the dough out onto a floured surface and knead gently a few times. Pat the dough into a 1•inch thick round.

7. Use a biscuit cutter to cut out rounds of dough and place them on a baking sheet lined with parchment paper.

8. Bake for 12•15 minutes or until the shortcakes are golden brown. Let the shortcakes cool slightly before assembling.

10. To assemble, slice the shortcakes in half horizontally. Spoon some strawberries and their juices onto the bottom half of each shortcake. Top with a dollop of whipped cream and place the other half of the shortcake on top. Serve the strawberry shortcakes immediately and enjoy!

This Strawberry Shortcake recipe is a delightful dessert that showcases the sweetness of fresh strawberries and the buttery richness of the shortcake. It's a perfect treat for any occasion!

# 89. Blueberry Muffins

**Ingredient:**

• 1 1/2 cups all•purpose flour
• 1/2 cup almond flour
• 1/4 cup sugar
• 1 tablespoon baking powder
• 1/4 teaspoon salt
• 1/2 cup unsweetened applesauce
• 1/4 cup low•fat milk
• 2 large eggs
• 1 teaspoon vanilla extract
• 1 cup fresh blueberries

**Instructions**:

1. Preheat the oven to 375°F (190°C) and line a muffin tin with paper liners.

2. In a mixing bowl, combine the all•purpose flour, almond flour, sugar, baking powder, and salt.

3. In a separate bowl, whisk together the unsweetened applesauce, low•fat milk, eggs, and vanilla extract.

4. Pour the wet ingredients into the dry ingredients and mix until just combined.

5. Gently fold in the fresh blueberries.

6. Divide the batter evenly among the muffin cups.

7. Bake the muffins in the preheated oven for about 18•20 minutes, or until a toothpick inserted into the center comes out clean.

8. Allow the muffins to cool in the tin for a few minutes before transferring them to a wire rack to cool completely.

These kidney•friendly Blueberry Muffins are a delicious and nutritious treat for seniors over 60 following a renal diet. The use of almond flour adds a nutty flavor and extra protein, while the fresh blueberries provide natural sweetness and antioxidants. Enjoy these muffins as a wholesome snack or breakfast option!

# 90. Chocolate Avocado Mousse

## Ingredient:

- 2 ripe avocados
- 1/4 cup unsweetened cocoa powder
- 1/4 cup honey or maple syrup
- 1 teaspoon vanilla extract
- 1/4 cup low•fat milk
- Optional toppings: sliced almonds, fresh berries

## Instructions:

1. Cut the avocados in half, remove the pits, and scoop out the flesh into a blender or food processor.

2. Add the unsweetened cocoa powder, honey or maple syrup, vanilla extract, and low•fat milk to the blender.

3. Blend the mixture until smooth and creamy, scraping down the sides as needed.

4. Taste the mousse and adjust the sweetness if needed by adding more honey or maple syrup.

5. Divide the chocolate avocado mousse into serving dishes or ramekins.

6. Chill the mousse in the refrigerator for at least 30 minutes before serving.

7. Garnish with sliced almonds and fresh berries if desired.

This Chocolate Avocado Mousse is a kidney•friendly dessert option for seniors over 60 following a renal diet. The avocado provides a creamy texture and healthy fats, while the cocoa powder adds a rich chocolate flavor without added sugar. Enjoy this decadent mousse as a guilt•free treat that is both delicious and nutritious!

# 91. Banana Oat Cookies

## Ingredient:

• 2 ripe bananas, mashed
• 1 1/2 cups old•fashioned oats
• 1/4 cup chopped nuts (such as walnuts or almonds)
• 1/4 cup raisins or dried cranberries
• 1/2 teaspoon cinnamon
• 1/4 teaspoon nutmeg
• 1/4 teaspoon salt
• 1 tablespoon honey or maple syrup (optional)

## Instructions:

1. Preheat the oven to 350°F (175°C) and line a baking sheet with parchment paper.

2. In a mixing bowl, combine the mashed bananas, old•fashioned oats, chopped nuts, raisins or dried cranberries, cinnamon, nutmeg, salt, and honey or maple syrup (if using). Mix well to combine.

3. Drop spoonfuls of the cookie dough onto the prepared baking sheet, spacing them apart.

4. Flatten each cookie slightly with the back of a spoon.

5. Bake the cookies in the preheated oven for about 15•20 minutes, or until golden brown.

6. Remove the cookies from the oven and let them cool on the baking sheet for a few minutes before transferring them to a wire rack to cool completely.

These Banana Oat Cookies are a kidney•friendly and nutritious snack option for seniors over 60 following a renal diet. The natural sweetness of bananas and optional honey or maple syrup provides a touch of sweetness without added sugar. Enjoy these wholesome cookies as a satisfying treat that is easy to make and delicious to enjoy!

# 92. Low•Sodium Cheesecake

## Ingredient:

### *For the Crust:*
• 1 1/2 cups graham cracker crumbs (look for low•sodium graham crackers)
• 1/4 cup unsalted butter, melted
• 1 tablespoon honey or maple syrup

### For the Cheesecake Filling:
• 16 oz low•sodium cream cheese, softened
• 1/2 cup low•fat Greek yogurt
• 1/2 cup sugar substitute (such as stevia or erythritol)
• 2 large eggs
• 1 teaspoon vanilla extract
• Zest of 1 lemon
• 1 tablespoon all•purpose flour

## Instructions:
1. Preheat the oven to 325°F (165°C) and grease a 9•inch springform pan.

2. In a mixing bowl, combine the graham cracker crumbs, melted butter, and honey or maple syrup for the crust. Press the mixture into the bottom of the prepared springform pan.

3. In a separate bowl, beat the low•sodium cream cheese until smooth.

4. Add the low•fat Greek yogurt, sugar substitute, eggs, vanilla extract, lemon zest, and flour to the cream cheese. Mix until well combined and smooth.

5. Pour the cheesecake filling over the crust in the springform pan. Bake the cheesecake in the preheated oven for about 45•50 minutes, or until the center is set.

6. Turn off the oven and let the cheesecake cool in the oven with the door slightly ajar for about 1 hour. Remove the cheesecake from the oven and refrigerate for at least 4 hours or overnight before serving.

This Low•Sodium Cheesecake is a kidney•friendly dessert option for seniors over 60 following a renal diet. The use of low•sodium ingredients and a sugar substitute helps reduce sodium and sugar content while still providing a delicious and creamy cheesecake experience. Enjoy a slice of this guilt•free treat for a special occasion or as a delightful dessert!

# 93. Mango Sorbet

## Ingredient:

• 2 ripe mangoes, peeled and diced
• 1/4 cup honey or maple syrup (optional)
• 1/4 cup water
• 1 tablespoon fresh lime juice
• 1/2 teaspoon vanilla extract

## Instructions:

1. Place the diced mangoes in a blender or food processor.

2. Add honey or maple syrup (if using), water, lime juice, and vanilla extract to the blender.

3. Blend the mixture until smooth and well combined.

4. Pour the mango mixture into a shallow dish or container suitable for freezing.

5. Place the dish in the freezer and let it freeze for about 2•3 hours.

6. Every 30 minutes, take the dish out of the freezer and stir the mixture with a fork to break up any ice crystals. Repeat this process until the sorbet is frozen and has a smooth texture.

7. Once the sorbet is ready, scoop it into serving dishes and enjoy!

This kidney•friendly Mango Sorbet is a refreshing and naturally sweet dessert option for seniors over 60 following a renal diet. The use of ripe mangoes provides a burst of tropical flavor, while the optional honey or maple syrup adds a touch of sweetness. Enjoy this sorbet as a light and satisfying treat on a warm day!

# 94. Pumpkin Pie (Low Sugar)

## Ingredient:

### For the Pumpkin Pie Filling:
• 1 can (15 oz) pumpkin puree
• 2 large eggs
• 1/2 cup low•fat milk
• 1/4 cup honey or maple syrup
• 1 teaspoon ground cinnamon
• 1/2 teaspoon ground ginger
• 1/4 teaspoon ground nutmeg
• 1/4 teaspoon salt

### For the Pie Crust:
• 1 pre•made low•sugar graham cracker crust or a homemade low•sugar pie crust

## Instructions:

1. Preheat the oven to 350°F (175°C).

2. In a mixing bowl, whisk together the pumpkin puree, eggs, low•fat milk, honey or maple syrup, cinnamon, ginger, nutmeg, and salt until well combined.

3. Pour the pumpkin pie filling into the pre•made graham cracker crust or homemade pie crust.

4. Bake the pie in the preheated oven for about 45•50 minutes, or until the filling is set.

5. Remove the pie from the oven and let it cool completely before serving.

This Low•Sugar Pumpkin Pie is a kidney•friendly dessert option for seniors over 60 following a renal diet. The use of pumpkin puree and warm spices like cinnamon, ginger, and nutmeg provides a comforting and flavorful pie without excessive sugar. Enjoy a slice of this delicious pumpkin pie as a special treat during the fall season or any time of the year!

# 95. Pineapple Upside•Down Cake

## Ingredient:

### For the Cake:
• 1 1/2 cups all•purpose flour
• 1/2 cup almond flour
• 1/2 cup sugar
• 1/4 cup unsweetened applesauce
• 1/4 cup low•fat milk
• 2 large eggs
• 1 teaspoon vanilla extract
• 1 teaspoon baking powder
• 1/4 teaspoon salt

### For the Pineapple Topping:
• 1 can (20 oz) pineapple slices in juice, drained
• 1/4 cup unsalted butter
• 1/2 cup brown sugar
• Maraschino cherries for garnish (optional)

## Instructions:

1. Preheat the oven to 350°F (175°C) and grease a 9•inch round cake pan.

2. In the cake pan, melt the unsalted butter and sprinkle the brown sugar evenly over the melted butter.

3. Arrange the drained pineapple slices on top of the brown sugar, placing a maraschino cherry in the center of each pineapple slice if desired.

4. In a mixing bowl, combine the all•purpose flour, almond flour, sugar, unsweetened applesauce, low•fat milk, eggs, vanilla extract, baking powder, and salt. Mix until well combined.

5. Pour the cake batter over the pineapple slices in the cake pan, spreading it evenly.

6. Bake the cake in the preheated oven for about 30•35 minutes, or until a toothpick inserted into the center comes out clean.  Allow the cake to cool in the pan for 10 minutes before inverting it onto a serving plate.

This kidney•friendly Pineapple Upside•Down Cake is a delicious and comforting dessert option for seniors over 60 following a renal diet. The use of almond flour adds a nutty flavor and texture, while the natural sweetness of pineapple and a touch of brown sugar provide a delightful treat without excessive sodium. Enjoy a slice of this classic cake as a special treat for any occasion!

# 96. Lemon Bars

## Ingredient:

### *For the Crust:*
• 1 cup all•purpose flour
• 1/2 cup unsalted butter, softened
• 1/4 cup powdered sugar
• Pinch of salt

### *For the Lemon Filling:*
• 1 cup granulated sugar
• 2 tablespoons all•purpose flour
• 1/2 teaspoon baking powder
• 2 large eggs
• 1/4 cup fresh lemon juice
• Zest of 1 lemon
• Powdered sugar for dusting

## Instructions:

1. Preheat the oven to 350°F (175°C) and grease an 8x8•inch baking pan.

2. In a mixing bowl, combine the flour, softened butter, powdered sugar, and salt for the crust. Mix until crumbly.

3. Press the crust mixture into the bottom of the prepared baking pan.

4. Bake the crust in the preheated oven for about 15•20 minutes, or until lightly golden.

5. While the crust is baking, prepare the lemon filling. In a separate bowl, whisk together the granulated sugar, flour, and baking powder.

6. Add the eggs, lemon juice, and lemon zest to the sugar mixture and whisk until well combined.

7. Pour the lemon filling over the baked crust.

8. Return the pan to the oven and bake for an additional 20•25 minutes, or until the filling is set. Allow the lemon bars to cool completely in the pan. Once cooled, dust the top with powdered sugar. Cut into squares and serve.

These Lemon Bars are a perfect balance of sweet and tangy, with a buttery crust and a zesty lemon filling. They make a delightful treat for any occasion!

# 97. Low•Sodium Brownies

**Ingredient:**

• 1/2 cup unsweetened applesauce
• 1/4 cup unsweetened cocoa powder
• 1/2 cup all•purpose flour
• 1/2 cup sugar substitute (such as stevia or erythritol)
• 1/4 teaspoon salt
• 1/4 teaspoon baking powder
• 1/4 cup chopped nuts (such as walnuts or almonds), optional

**Instructions:**

1. Preheat the oven to 350°F (175°C) and grease an 8x8•inch baking pan.

2. In a mixing bowl, combine the unsweetened applesauce and unsweetened cocoa powder until smooth.

3. Add the all•purpose flour, sugar substitute, salt, and baking powder to the applesauce mixture. Mix until well combined.

4. If using chopped nuts, fold them into the brownie batter.

5. Pour the brownie batter into the prepared baking pan and spread it evenly.

6. Bake the brownies in the preheated oven for about 20•25 minutes, or until a toothpick inserted into the center comes out clean.

7. Allow the brownies to cool in the pan before cutting them into squares.

These Low•Sodium Brownies are a kidney•friendly dessert option for seniors over 60 following a renal diet. The use of unsweetened applesauce and a sugar substitute helps reduce sodium and sugar content while still providing a satisfying and chocolatey treat. Enjoy these brownies as a guilt•free indulgence that is both delicious and suitable for a renal diet.

# 98. Raspberry Sorbet

## Ingredient:

• 4 cups fresh or frozen raspberries
• 1/2 cup water
• 1/4 cup honey or sugar substitute
• 1 tablespoon lemon juice

## Instructions:

1. In a blender or food processor, blend the raspberries until smooth.

2. Strain the raspberry puree through a fine mesh sieve to remove the seeds.

3. In a saucepan, combine the raspberry puree, water, honey (or sugar substitute), and lemon juice. Heat over medium heat until the mixture is well combined and slightly thickened.

4. Remove from heat and let the mixture cool to room temperature.

5. Pour the mixture into a shallow dish and place it in the freezer.

6. Every 30 minutes, stir the mixture with a fork to break up any ice crystals. Repeat this process until the sorbet is frozen and has a smooth consistency.

7. Serve the raspberry sorbet in small bowls or cones and enjoy!

This raspberry sorbet is a refreshing and kidney•friendly dessert option for seniors following a renal diet. Remember to consult with a healthcare provider or a dietitian to ensure it fits within individual dietary restrictions and needs.

# 99. Coconut Macaroons

**Ingredient:**

• 3 cups shredded coconut
• 3/4 cup sweetened condensed milk
• 1 teaspoon vanilla extract
• 2 large egg whites
• 1/4 teaspoon salt

**Instructions:**

1. Preheat your oven to 325°F (165°C) and line a baking sheet with parchment paper.

2. In a mixing bowl, combine the shredded coconut, sweetened condensed milk, and vanilla extract. Mix well until all ingredients are evenly incorporated.

3. In a separate clean bowl, beat the egg whites and salt until stiff peaks form.

4. Gently fold the beaten egg whites into the coconut mixture until well combined.

5. Using a spoon or cookie scoop, drop rounded tablespoons of the mixture onto the prepared baking sheet, spacing them about an inch apart.

6. Bake in the preheated oven for about 20•25 minutes, or until the macaroons are golden brown on the outside.

7. Allow the macaroons to cool on the baking sheet for a few minutes before transferring them to a wire rack to cool completely.

These coconut macaroons are sweet, chewy, and perfect for a delightful treat. Enjoy them with a cup of tea or coffee, or share them with family and friends.

# 100. Berry Tart with Almond Crust

## Ingredient:

### *For the Almond Crust:*
• 1 cup almond flour
• 1/4 cup unsalted butter, melted
• 2 tablespoons honey or maple syrup
• 1/4 teaspoon salt

### *For the Berry Filling:*
• 2 cups mixed berries (such as strawberries, blueberries, raspberries)
• 1/4 cup honey or maple syrup
• 1 tablespoon cornstarch
• 1/4 cup water
• 1 teaspoon vanilla extract

## Instructions:
1. Preheat the oven to 350°F (180°C).

2. In a bowl, mix together the almond flour, melted butter, honey or maple syrup, and salt until well combined.

3. Press the almond mixture into a tart pan, covering the bottom and sides evenly.

4. Bake the almond crust in the preheated oven for about 10•12 minutes, or until lightly golden. Remove from the oven and let it cool.

5. In a saucepan, combine the mixed berries, honey or maple syrup, cornstarch, water, and vanilla extract.

6. Cook the berry mixture over medium heat, stirring occasionally, until the berries soften and the mixture thickens slightly. Remove the berry filling from heat and let it cool slightly.

7. Pour the berry filling into the cooled almond crust. Chill the berry tart in the refrigerator for at least 1•2 hours before serving.

This kidney•friendly Berry Tart with Almond Crust is a delightful and nutritious dessert option for seniors over 60 following a renal diet. The almond crust adds a nutty flavor and texture, while the mixed berries provide natural sweetness and a burst of color. Enjoy this delicious tart as a special treat for any occasion!

# 101. Chocolate•Dipped Strawberries

**Ingredient:**

• Fresh strawberries
• Dark chocolate (with lower potassium content if needed)
• Chopped nuts (optional)

**Instructions:**

1. Wash the strawberries thoroughly and pat them dry with a paper towel.

2. In a microwave•safe bowl, melt the dark chocolate in short intervals, stirring in between until smooth.

3. Dip each strawberry into the melted chocolate, coating it halfway or fully as desired.

4. Place the chocolate•dipped strawberries on a parchment•lined tray.

5. If using chopped nuts, sprinkle them over the chocolate before it sets.

6. Allow the chocolate to set by placing the tray in the refrigerator for about 15•20 minutes.

7. Once the chocolate is firm, the chocolate•dipped strawberries are ready to be enjoyed.

These Chocolate•Dipped Strawberries are a delicious and kidney•friendly dessert option for seniors following a renal diet. Dark chocolate is lower in potassium compared to milk chocolate, making it a better choice for those with dietary restrictions. Enjoy these sweet treats as a special indulgence or share them with loved ones for a delightful and healthy dessert experience.

# 102. Orange Gelatin with Whipped Cream

**Ingredient:**

• 1 package of sugar•free orange gelatin mix
• 1 cup boiling water
• 1 cup cold water
• Whipped cream (made with low•fat or non•dairy options)

**Instructions**:

1. In a mixing bowl, dissolve the sugar•free orange gelatin mix in 1 cup of boiling water, stirring until completely dissolved.

2. Stir in 1 cup of cold water into the gelatin mixture.

3. Pour the gelatin mixture into individual serving cups or a large serving dish.

4. Refrigerate the gelatin for at least 4 hours, or until set.

5. Once the gelatin is set, top each serving with a dollop of whipped cream.

6. Serve the Orange Gelatin with Whipped Cream chilled and enjoy!

This Orange Gelatin with Whipped Cream is a light and refreshing dessert that is low in potassium and suitable for a renal diet for seniors over 60. The sugar•free orange gelatin provides a burst of citrus flavor, while the whipped cream adds a creamy and indulgent touch. This dessert is easy to prepare and can be a satisfying treat for those looking for a kidney•friendly option.

# 103. Carrot Cake (Low Sugar)

## Ingredient:

- 2 cups grated carrots
- 1/2 cup unsweetened applesauce
- 1/4 cup vegetable oil
- 2 eggs
- 1 teaspoon vanilla extract
- 1 cup all•purpose flour
- 1/2 cup whole wheat flour
- 1 teaspoon baking soda
- 1/2 teaspoon baking powder
- 1/2 teaspoon salt
- 1 teaspoon ground cinnamon
- 1/4 teaspoon ground nutmeg
- 1/4 cup chopped walnuts or pecans (optional)
- Cream cheese frosting (optional)

## Instructions:

1. Preheat your oven to 350°F (175°C) and grease a cake pan.

2. In a mixing bowl, combine the grated carrots, applesauce, vegetable oil, eggs, and vanilla extract. Mix well.

3. In a separate bowl, whisk together the all•purpose flour, whole wheat flour, baking soda, baking powder, salt, cinnamon, and nutmeg.

4. Gradually add the dry ingredients to the wet ingredients, stirring until just combined.
5. Fold in the chopped nuts, if using.

6. Pour the batter into the prepared cake pan and spread it out evenly.

7. Bake in the preheated oven for about 25•30 minutes, or until a toothpick inserted into the center comes out clean.

8. Allow the carrot cake to cool in the pan before removing it and transferring it to a wire rack to cool completely. Optionally, frost the cooled cake with a thin layer of cream cheese frosting.

This Low•Sugar Carrot Cake is a healthier version of the classic dessert, with the natural sweetness of carrots and applesauce reducing the need for added sugar. Enjoy a slice of this moist and flavorful cake as a guilt•free treat. The addition of nuts provides a crunchy texture and extra flavor. Feel free to customize the cake with your favorite frosting or enjoy it as is for a delicious and satisfying dessert.

# 104. Pear and Ginger Compote

**Ingredient:**

• 4 ripe pears, peeled, cored, and diced
• 1/4 cup water
• 2 tablespoons honey or sugar substitute
• 1 teaspoon fresh ginger, grated
• 1/2 teaspoon ground cinnamon
• 1/4 teaspoon ground nutmeg
• 1/4 teaspoon vanilla extract

**Instructions:**

1. In a saucepan, combine the diced pears, water, honey (or sugar substitute), grated ginger, cinnamon, and nutmeg.

2. Cook the mixture over medium heat, stirring occasionally, until the pears are tender and the liquid has thickened to a syrup•like consistency.

3. Remove the saucepan from heat and stir in the vanilla extract.

4. Allow the Pear and Ginger Compote to cool slightly before serving.

This Pear and Ginger Compote is a warm and comforting dessert that combines the natural sweetness of pears with the warmth of ginger and spices. The addition of ginger adds a subtle kick and depth of flavor to the compote. Enjoy this kidney•friendly dessert on its own or as a topping for yogurt, oatmeal, or ice cream. It's a delicious and nutritious treat that can be enjoyed by seniors over 60 as part of a renal diet.

# 105. Low•Sodium Sugar Cookies

**Ingredient:**

• 2 cups all•purpose flour
• 1/2 teaspoon baking powder
• 1/4 teaspoon salt (or omit salt for even lower sodium)
• 1/2 cup unsalted butter, softened
• 3/4 cup granulated sugar
• 1 large egg
• 1 teaspoon vanilla extract

**Instructions:**

1. Preheat your oven to 350°F (175°C) and line a baking sheet with parchment paper.

2. In a medium bowl, whisk together the flour, baking powder, and salt (if using).

3. In a separate large bowl, cream together the softened butter and sugar until light and fluffy.

4. Beat in the egg and vanilla extract until well combined.

5. Gradually add the dry ingredients to the wet ingredients, mixing until a dough forms.

6. Roll the dough into small balls and place them on the prepared baking sheet, spacing them a few inches apart.

7. Flatten each ball slightly with the bottom of a glass or fork.

8. Bake in the preheated oven for about 8•10 minutes, or until the edges are lightly golden.

9. Allow the cookies to cool on the baking sheet for a few minutes before transferring them to a wire rack to cool completely.

These low•sodium sugar cookies are a delicious and healthier option for those watching their sodium intake. Feel free to customize them by adding a sprinkle of cinnamon or a touch of lemon zest for extra flavor. Enjoy these cookies as a tasty treat without the high sodium content.

# 106. Coconut Rice Pudding

## Ingredient:

• 1 cup jasmine rice
• 2 cups water
• 1 can (13.5 oz) coconut milk
• 1/2 cup sugar
• 1/2 teaspoon salt
• 1 teaspoon vanilla extract
• 1/2 cup shredded coconut (optional)
• Ground cinnamon for garnish

## Instructions:

1. In a saucepan, combine the jasmine rice and water. Bring to a boil, then reduce heat, cover, and simmer for about 15•20 minutes, or until the rice is cooked and the water is absorbed.

2. Stir in the coconut milk, sugar, salt, and vanilla extract. Cook over low heat, stirring occasionally, for another 15•20 minutes, or until the mixture thickens to a pudding•like consistency.

3. If using shredded coconut, stir it into the rice pudding.

4. Remove the rice pudding from heat and let it cool slightly.

5. Serve the coconut rice pudding warm or chilled, garnished with a sprinkle of ground cinnamon.

This Coconut Rice Pudding is a creamy and comforting dessert with a tropical twist. The combination of coconut milk and shredded coconut adds a rich and flavorful touch to the classic rice pudding. Enjoy this sweet treat as a delicious ending to a meal or as a satisfying snack.

# 107. Apple Turnovers

## Ingredient:

• 2 large apples, peeled, cored, and diced
• 1/4 cup granulated sugar
• 1 teaspoon ground cinnamon
• 1/4 teaspoon ground nutmeg
• 1 tablespoon lemon juice
• 1 tablespoon cornstarch
• 1 package of puff pastry sheets, thawed
• 1 egg, beaten (for egg wash)
• Powdered sugar for dusting (optional)

## Instructions:

1. Preheat your oven to 400°F (200°C) and line a baking sheet with parchment paper.

2. In a bowl, combine the diced apples, granulated sugar, cinnamon, nutmeg, lemon juice, and cornstarch. Mix well to coat the apples evenly.

3. Roll out the puff pastry sheets on a lightly floured surface and cut each sheet into squares.

4. Place a spoonful of the apple mixture onto one half of each pastry square, leaving a border around the edges.

5. Fold the other half of the pastry over the apple filling to create a triangle shape. Use a fork to crimp the edges and seal the turnovers.

6. Brush the tops of the turnovers with the beaten egg for a golden finish.

7. Place the turnovers on the prepared baking sheet and bake in the preheated oven for about 20•25 minutes, or until the pastry is golden brown and crispy.

8. Allow the apple turnovers to cool slightly before serving. Dust with powdered sugar if desired.

These Apple Turnovers are a delicious and flaky pastry filled with sweet and spiced apple filling. Enjoy them as a delightful dessert or a special treat with a cup of tea or coffee. The warm and comforting flavors of the apple turnovers make them a perfect indulgence for any time of the day.

# 108. Cranberry Oat Bars

## Ingredient:

• 1 cup all•purpose flour
• 1 cup old•fashioned oats
• 1/2 cup brown sugar
• 1/4 teaspoon baking soda
• 1/4 teaspoon salt
• 1/2 cup unsalted butter, melted
• 1 cup cranberry sauce (homemade or store•bought)

## Instructions:

1. Preheat your oven to 350°F (175°C) and grease or line an 8x8•inch baking pan with parchment paper.

2. In a mixing bowl, combine the flour, oats, brown sugar, baking soda, and salt.

3. Add the melted butter to the dry ingredients and mix until well combined and crumbly.

4. Press two•thirds of the oat mixture into the bottom of the prepared baking pan to form the base.

5. Spread the cranberry sauce evenly over the oat base.

6. Sprinkle the remaining oat mixture over the cranberry layer as a crumble topping.

7. Bake in the preheated oven for about 25•30 minutes, or until the top is golden brown.

8. Allow the cranberry oat bars to cool in the pan before cutting them into squares.

These Cranberry Oat Bars are a delicious and wholesome treat that combines the tartness of cranberries with the sweetness of oats. Enjoy them as a snack or dessert, and feel free to customize the recipe by adding nuts or spices like cinnamon for extra flavor.

# 109. Banana Bread (Low Potassium)

## Ingredient:

- 2 ripe bananas, mashed
- 1/3 cup unsweetened applesauce
- 1/4 cup low•fat milk
- 1/4 cup vegetable oil
- 1 teaspoon vanilla extract
- 1 1/2 cups all•purpose flour
- 1/2 cup granulated sugar
- 1 teaspoon baking powder
- 1/2 teaspoon baking soda
- 1/4 teaspoon salt
- 1/2 teaspoon ground cinnamon
- 1/4 cup chopped walnuts (optional)

## Instructions:

1. Preheat your oven to 350°F (175°C) and grease a loaf pan.

2. In a mixing bowl, combine the mashed bananas, applesauce, milk, vegetable oil, and vanilla extract.

3. In a separate bowl, whisk together the flour, sugar, baking powder, baking soda, salt, and cinnamon.

4. Gradually add the dry ingredients to the wet ingredients, mixing until just combined. Be careful not to overmix.

5. Fold in the chopped walnuts, if using.

6. Pour the batter into the prepared loaf pan and spread it out evenly.

7. Bake in the preheated oven for about 50•60 minutes, or until a toothpick inserted into the center comes out clean.

8. Allow the banana bread to cool in the pan for 10 minutes before transferring it to a wire rack to cool completely.

This Low Potassium Banana Bread is a kidney•friendly option for seniors following a renal diet. By using ingredients low in potassium, such as applesauce instead of eggs and low•fat milk, this recipe reduces the potassium content while still maintaining the delicious flavor and texture of traditional banana bread. Enjoy a slice of this bread as a wholesome snack or breakfast treat.

# 110. Lemon Poppy Seed Cookies

**Ingredient:**

• 1 cup all•purpose flour
• 1/2 teaspoon baking powder
• 1/4 teaspoon salt
• Zest of 1 lemon
• 1 tablespoon poppy seeds
• 1/2 cup unsalted butter, softened
• 1/2 cup granulated sugar
• 1 egg
• 1 tablespoon fresh lemon juice
• 1/2 teaspoon vanilla extract

**Instructions:**
1. Preheat your oven to 350°F (175°C) and line a baking sheet with parchment paper.

2. In a bowl, whisk together the flour, baking powder, salt, lemon zest, and poppy seeds.

3. In a separate bowl, cream together the softened butter and sugar until light and fluffy.
4. Beat in the egg, lemon juice, and vanilla extract until well combined.

5. Gradually add the dry ingredients to the wet ingredients, mixing until a dough forms.

6. Drop rounded tablespoons of dough onto the prepared baking sheet, spacing them a few inches apart.

7. Flatten each cookie slightly with the back of a spoon or fork.

8. Bake in the preheated oven for about 10•12 minutes, or until the edges are lightly golden.

9. Allow the cookies to cool on the baking sheet for a few minutes before transferring them to a wire rack to cool completely.

These Lemon Poppy Seed Cookies are light, fragrant, and perfect for citrus lovers. The combination of lemon zest and poppy seeds gives these cookies a delightful flavor and texture. Enjoy them with a cup of tea or as a sweet treat any time of the day.

# 111. Fresh Melon Balls

**Ingredient:**

• Assorted melons (such as watermelon, cantaloupe, honeydew)
• Mint leaves for garnish (optional)

**Instructions:**
1. Wash the melons thoroughly under running water.

2. Cut the melons in half and scoop out the seeds.

3. Use a melon baller to scoop out small, round melon balls from the flesh of each melon.

4. Place the melon balls in a serving bowl or arrange them on a platter.

5. Garnish with fresh mint leaves for added flavor and presentation.

6. Serve the fresh melon balls immediately or chill them in the refrigerator before serving for a refreshing treat.

These Fresh Melon Balls are a simple and healthy snack that is perfect for hot summer days or as a light dessert option. Melons are hydrating, low in calories, and packed with vitamins and minerals, making them a nutritious choice for seniors over 60. Enjoy the natural sweetness and juiciness of the melon balls as a guilt•free treat any time of the day.

# 112. Blackberries with Greek Yogurt

**Ingredient:**

• Fresh blackberries
• Greek yogurt
• Honey or maple syrup (optional)
• Granola (optional)

**Instructions:**

1. Wash the blackberries thoroughly and pat them dry with a paper towel.

2. In a serving bowl or glass, spoon a generous portion of Greek yogurt.

3. Top the Greek yogurt with a handful of fresh blackberries.

4. Drizzle a little honey or maple syrup over the blackberries for added sweetness, if desired.

5. Optionally, sprinkle some granola on top for a crunchy texture and extra flavor.

6. Serve the blackberries with Greek yogurt immediately and enjoy!

This Blackberries with Greek Yogurt recipe is a quick and easy way to enjoy a healthy and satisfying snack or breakfast. The combination of creamy Greek yogurt with sweet and tangy blackberries creates a delicious contrast of flavors and textures. Feel free to customize this dish by adding nuts, seeds, or a sprinkle of cinnamon for extra taste and nutrition.

# 113. Pineapple Coconut Smoothie

**Ingredient:**

• 1 cup fresh or frozen pineapple chunks
• 1/2 cup coconut milk (unsweetened)
• 1/2 cup plain Greek yogurt (low•fat or non•fat)
• 1 tablespoon honey or sugar substitute (optional)
• Ice cubes (optional)

**Instructions:**

1. In a blender, combine the pineapple chunks, coconut milk, Greek yogurt, and honey (if using).

2. Blend the ingredients until smooth and well combined. If you prefer a thicker consistency, you can add some ice cubes and blend again.

3. Taste the smoothie and adjust the sweetness if needed by adding more honey or sugar substitute.

4. Pour the Pineapple Coconut Smoothie into a glass and serve chilled.

This Pineapple Coconut Smoothie is a refreshing and kidney•friendly beverage that is low in sodium and can be a nutritious addition to a renal diet for seniors over 60. Pineapple adds natural sweetness, while coconut milk provides a creamy texture and flavor. Greek yogurt adds protein and creaminess to the smoothie. Enjoy this tropical treat as a snack or a light meal.

# 114. Strawberry Rhubarb Crisp

## Ingredient:

### For the Topping:
• 1 cup old•fashioned oats
• 1/2 cup all•purpose flour
• 1/2 cup brown sugar
• 1/2 teaspoon ground cinnamon
• 1/4 teaspoon salt
• 1/2 cup unsalted butter, melted

### For the Filling:
• 2 cups chopped rhubarb
• 2 cups sliced strawberries
• 1/2 cup granulated sugar
• 2 tablespoons cornstarch
• 1 teaspoon vanilla extract

## Instructions:

1. Preheat your oven to 350°F (175°C) and grease a baking dish.

2. In a large bowl, combine the chopped rhubarb, sliced strawberries, granulated sugar, cornstarch, and vanilla extract. Mix well to coat the fruit evenly.

3. Pour the fruit mixture into the prepared baking dish, spreading it out into an even layer.

4. In another bowl, combine the oats, flour, brown sugar, cinnamon, and salt for the topping.

5. Pour the melted butter over the oat mixture and stir until it resembles coarse crumbs.

6. Sprinkle the oat topping evenly over the fruit mixture in the baking dish.

7. Bake in the preheated oven for about 35•40 minutes, or until the fruit is bubbly and the topping is golden brown.

8. Allow the crisp to cool slightly before serving. Enjoy warm with a scoop of vanilla ice cream or a dollop of whipped cream, if desired.

This Strawberry Rhubarb Crisp is a delightful dessert that captures the flavors of spring and summer. The combination of sweet strawberries and tangy rhubarb, topped with a crunchy oat topping, makes for a perfect treat. Enjoy this crisp on its own or with your favorite accompaniment for a delicious dessert experience.

# 115. Cinnamon Apple Chips

## Ingredient:

• 2•3 large apples (such as Granny Smith or Honeycrisp)
• 1•2 teaspoons ground cinnamon
• Optional: a sprinkle of sugar or sugar substitute

## Instructions:

1. Preheat your oven to 200°F (95°C) and line a baking sheet with parchment paper.

2. Wash and thinly slice the apples using a sharp knife or a mandoline slicer, removing the seeds and core.

3. In a bowl, toss the apple slices with ground cinnamon until they are evenly coated. You can also add a sprinkle of sugar or sugar substitute if desired.

4. Place the apple slices in a single layer on the prepared baking sheet, making sure they do not overlap.

5. Bake in the preheated oven for about 1.5 to 2 hours, flipping the slices halfway through the baking time.

6. Keep an eye on the apple chips towards the end of the baking time to prevent them from burning. The chips are done when they are crisp and slightly golden.

7. Remove the apple chips from the oven and let them cool completely before enjoying.

These homemade Cinnamon Apple Chips are a healthy and flavorful snack that is perfect for satisfying your sweet cravings. Store any leftovers in an airtight container to maintain their crispness. Enjoy these apple chips as a tasty and nutritious treat!

As we come to the end of the ***"Renal Diet Cookbook for Seniors Over 60: Supporting Your Kidneys with Wholesome, Balanced Meals,"*** *we hope you feel equipped and inspired to take control of your kidney health through thoughtful and delicious nutrition. The journey of managing kidney disease can be challenging, but with the right knowledge and tools, it is entirely possible to lead a fulfilling and healthy life.*

*Throughout this book, we have explored the importance of kidney health and how a balanced diet can play a pivotal role in managing and supporting renal function. We've provided you with essential nutritional guidelines, practical meal planning advice, and a variety of recipes that prove kidney-friendly meals can be both nutritious and enjoyable.*

*Remember, the key to a successful renal diet lies in consistency and variety. By incorporating the recipes and tips from this cookbook into your daily routine, you are taking proactive steps toward better health and well-being. Each meal is an opportunity to nourish your body and support your kidneys, and with the delicious options provided, you can do so without compromising on taste or satisfaction.*

*We encourage you to continue experimenting with the recipes, adjusting them to suit your preferences, and exploring new ingredients that align with your dietary needs. Don't hesitate to share your culinary creations with friends and family—good food is meant to be enjoyed together.*

*In addition to following a kidney-friendly diet, remember to stay hydrated, keep active, and consult with your healthcare provider regularly to monitor your health and adjust your dietary plan as needed. Your journey to better kidney health is ongoing, and every small step you take contributes to a larger, healthier lifestyle.*

*Thank you for allowing this cookbook to be a part of your journey. We hope it has provided you with valuable insights, practical tools, and a renewed sense of confidence in managing your kidney health. May your days be filled with vitality, joy, and the pleasure of wholesome, balanced meals.*

*Here's to your continued health and happiness!*

*Warmest regards,*